We Know How This Ends

We Know How This Ends

Living while Dying

Bruce H. Kramer
with Cathy Wurzer

University of Minnesota Press
Minneapolis | London

Portions of this book first appeared on Bruce Kramer's blog, Dis Ease
Diary.

Published by the University of Minnesota Press
111 Third Avenue South, Suite 290
Minneapolis, MN 55401–2520
http://www.upress.umn.edu

Library of Congress Cataloging-in-Publication Data
Kramer, Bruce H.
We know how this ends : living while dying / Bruce H. Kramer; with
Cathy Wurzer.
ISBN 978-0-8166-9733-5 (hc)
1. Kramer, Bruce H.—Health. 2. Amyotropic lateral sclerosis—
Patients—United States—Biography. I. Wurzer, Cathy. II. Title.
RC406.A24K73 2015
362.1968390092—dc23 [B]   2015000049

Printed in the United States of America on acid-free paper

The University of Minnesota is an equal-opportunity educator
and employer.

21 20 19 18 17 16 15   10 9 8 7 6 5 4 3 2 1

This book is dedicated to Evelyn Emerson,
Bruce's muse and one true love;
to Fritz Wurzer, Cathy's father, who taught her
many lessons about living and dying;
and to all those who suffer and have yet to find their way.

CONTENTS

PROLOGUE

Cathy Wurzer

The request reflected the stark and sharply cold day outside. It was delivered with an understated urgency as a column of brilliant sunlight illuminated the small den.

"I'd like you to deliver the eulogy at my funeral."

The request was simple and should not have come as a surprise, but the words, and what they meant, made my stomach clutch. I was trying to find my breath and the right words to say, all at the same time.

Bruce Kramer sat quietly and waited for an answer. Waiting is what Bruce is forced to do. His motionless hands were placed carefully on each thigh. Swollen fingers often involuntarily cramp and curl if not straightened by a caregiver. His body, once sleek and athletic, is unraveling muscle by muscle and is now virtually paralyzed, unable to move on its own.

I couldn't look at Bruce. Instead I watched bare tree branches that were swaying back and forth in that afternoon's cold wind. My only thought was "My God, is Bruce telling me he is going to die soon?"

Bruce Kramer is dying, and dying as if in slow motion, because of a brutal illness that has a deceptively simple three-letter moniker: ALS. The full name of the incurable killer is amyotrophic lateral sclerosis. It is a relentless disease that worsens over time as the neurons in the brain and spinal cord mysteriously stop communicating with the body's muscles. Not only is physical movement affected but so are talking, swallowing, and breathing.

There is no cure for ALS. Most people who have ALS die in two to five years. Bruce is now in his fourth year after having been "reborn and baptized with the holy gifts of ALS." He wrote that memorable description on the first anniversary of his diagnosis in a blog that he has kept regularly about his life with ALS, begun only a few months after his diagnosis in December 2010. Since then, as a broadcast journalist, I have spent more than three years with Bruce crafting a series of recorded conversations for Minnesota Public Radio and its website, mprnews.org, about his experience of living with ALS. We have talked about the gifts and lessons of living with a terminal illness, both in private discussions and in conversations with a worldwide reach. The response to the series has been profound and universally positive; many people say they see their own lives reflected in Bruce's experiences even if they are not dealing with terminal illness. This book is based on Bruce's blog and on those forthright conversations.

Our professional relationship actually predates Bruce's experience with ALS. An accomplished musician and part-time church choir director, Bruce had helped arrange traditional Christian hymns with a local Indonesian gamelan group that uses gongs and other percussive instruments to perform its exotic melodies. Bruce and I did an interview in 2008 about his work, which was a cross-cultural musical delight that made for a wonderful four minutes of radio airtime. Bruce, at the time a dean at the University of St. Thomas in Minneapolis, provided a fascinating and engaging interview. It was a fun story, then I quickly forgot about him and the gamelan ensemble.

Bruce reentered my life in 2011. I had heard through a mutual friend that he had been diagnosed with ALS and had been blogging about his experiences. What struck me as I read the blog was how Bruce shied away from the mundane and instead dug deeper and wrote eloquently about the larger philosophical issues reflected in his disease. He was bluntly honest—in one blog he wrote, "I am no saint and I am pissed." Who wouldn't be angry in a similar situation?

Another mutual friend thought a series of broadcast conversations with Bruce about his life with ALS would be interesting, given his expressive and thoughtful nature. I was reluctant at first. At the time, my own life was filled with heartbreak because of disease, disability, and a decaying marriage, and I hesitated to explore someone else's pain. I had sick and aging parents who lived a couple of hours away, and I was juggling their changing circumstances with challenging ones of my own.

When we finally sat down to talk, that first radio segment included a few references to following Bruce "on his journey with ALS." I thought this was an apt metaphor, not only for what Bruce and his family were going through but also to describe how I envisioned the series. No one knew how long the journey would take, and the road would be fraught with twists and turns—after all, isn't life like a highway? Well, no, insisted Bruce: "This isn't a journey, this is life."

That is a difficult lesson to learn, but Bruce is a master teacher. Even though teaching is in his DNA (with both parents, grandparents, and even his spouse being teachers), Bruce did not come to teaching willingly. He earned his education degree because his college counseled that if he did not make it as a music performer, he could always fall back on teaching. It wasn't until he stood before his first classroom of students that he recognized the profession as a vocation, a calling in the true sense of the word.

Journalism at its best also teaches. The finest practitioners of the craft can transport readers, listeners, and viewers—whether through a seventy-inch article or a ninety-second broadcast story—to another place, sparking deeper understanding of an event or issue. The length of the story doesn't matter: it's about the connection that it makes. Good storytelling, like good teaching, creates connections. Those connections can educate and enlighten.

We all need to tell stories. This story is about the inevitability of all-too-human bodies breaking down, of living while embracing death instead of disengaging and denying it. It is a story of great loss—but in loss, there can be transformation.

Think back to the miracle of metamorphosis first taught to us in grade school. Small yellow, black, and white striped caterpillars are left in a glass aquarium in a fourth- or fifth-grade classroom to dutifully play their role in what becomes an amazing transformation into striking orange and black butterflies. Young students learn that all lives, from insects to mammals, change, and sometimes the changes are dramatic.

The lessons extend far beyond fifth-grade science. In each loss we experience, there is change, and in loss there can be growth, even during life's final transformation, death, where the most profound lessons are taught. Each loss offers a teachable moment, and, as Bruce points out, in the teachable moment is "an opportunity to grow until growth is no longer possible, a road map to the ultimate outcome."

I have been avoiding the ultimate outcome. Most of us want to.

On that bleak and brutally cold winter afternoon, Bruce had a sad, resigned look as he tried to describe the feeling of winding down and the sense that death is inching closer. He was trying to get his affairs in order, and that included making sure I am willing to eulogize him at his funeral. He knows that as a broadcaster and a professional performer I have the ability to gracefully and effectively power through difficult circumstances; as he said, I won't "dissolve into a blubbering mess" at the church's lectern. Bruce is a no-nonsense guy.

I took what seemed like minutes to finally answer Bruce, but all I could muster was to nod numbly as tears started leaking from the corners of my eyes.

It is difficult to say no to Bruce Kramer.

As we grow older (or perhaps when death is at hand), it is natural to ponder the meaning of our life and to ask what might be the lasting effects of our time in this world. It's natural to want to leave behind a meaningful legacy. This book could be viewed as part of Bruce's legacy, but, as he wrote, "The difference here is legacy is an act of ego, while teaching is an act of faith." Bruce is first and foremost a teacher. Good teachers hope they make a difference in the lives of their students. Teachers practice this faith daily.

We have faith in how this ends, and that is the point of this book.

Whatever challenges you face now or will face in the future, the experiences related here go beyond any one person's life. They reflect the elements that make us engage with life on a deeper level and ultimately define us as the human beings we can become.

In the book *Letters to a Young Poet,* Rainer Maria Rilke writes: "Do not now seek the answers, which cannot be given you because you would not be able to live them. And the point is, to live everything. Live the questions now. Perhaps you will then gradually, without noticing it, live along some distant day into the answer."

Bruce Kramer has been living life's questions while he is dying.

What follows may offer some answers for us all.

I

PARALLEL LIVES

2010 was a great year. In no particular order, I completed my second year as dean of the College of Education, Leadership, and Counseling at the University of St. Thomas, my wife was happily teaching music in a French immersion elementary school, my sons were getting themselves together—each had found a life partner, and we knew it would be just a matter of time before they got married. We had two cats, I was a bike commuter, I rode the MS 150 to raise money for multiple sclerosis, Ev and I spent a month in Indonesia playing Indonesian gamelan music, and I lectured at two Indonesian universities. We drank a lot of wine, and we ate a lot of fish.

2010 was a great year.

Early in February 2010 I thought very little of the fasciculations that made my leg muscles dance and twitch on their own, especially when I was tired. I thought very little of the fall I experienced down a set of stairs in a parking garage. By April, I noticed that I needed to scoop my leg into the car with my left hand. It wasn't a big deal, and I thought it just had to do with the angle in which I was sitting, but the reality was I could not lift my leg without assistance from my hand.

By June, in Indonesia, I couldn't seem to shake an overarching feeling of fatigue, a jet lag that seemed kind of normal since I had just flown halfway around the world. But it wouldn't go away, and I spent the entire trip always a little tired, not myself. During this trip, Cathy Wurzer at Minnesota Public Radio interviewed me as spokesperson for our gamelan group. It was 6 a.m. in Minnesota and 6 p.m. in Java: we pulled our bus over to the side of the highway, and everyone sat quietly while I spoke with Cathy on the phone. I remember wondering how it came out on the other end, because I was so tired, but overall on that trip we had a great time.

In July we were walking the path around Lake Harriet. Evelyn observed, "Your foot sounds funny, it sounds like step kerflop, step kerflop." The following month I visited my fine general practitioner for my annual physical. At the end of her examination, she asked, "Anything else?"

"Well, yes. I have this floppy foot that doesn't respond, and I wonder what it is."

She watched me walk and suggested I have it checked by a neurologist. She gave me a referral, stating that it was probably "nothing more than a pinched nerve." I blew it off. I was fifty-four and healthy and saw no reason to take time out of my busy schedule to go to someone who would probably just tell me to do a little physical therapy.

Labor Day weekend Ev and I were on our annual last big bike ride of the year on the Root River Trail in southern Minnesota. It was our tradition to take a long ride on the Sunday prior to the holiday, pick up apples at an orchard in Preston on Monday, and arrive home in time to have family over for apple pie. The previous year, we had ridden one end of the trail to the other: eighty-six miles round-trip. This year, we decided we weren't in quite that condition, and settled on thirty miles out and thirty miles back as a good ride. Forty-five miles into the ride I could not keep up with her. Ev thought I was kidding, that I was trying to jolly her along on the last fifteen miles to encourage her. But I was not kidding. When we reached our bed-and-breakfast, I collapsed and slept.

I was beginning to notice on my morning and evening bike commutes that I couldn't pull with my left leg, even though I was clipped into the pedals. Spinning was becoming a joke. I really needed to take some time to get this pinched nerve, my sciatica, whatever it was, looked at.

October. We were preparing for a gamelan performance, sort of reliving the Indonesian tour we had taken in the summer. I was the emcee, and even though I was exhausted, I was happy to do it. I started down the stairs from the stage to the auditorium floor, and my leg gave out and sent me tumbling forward. I could not get up by myself; I was simply too weak. One week later, at a conference in New Orleans, I was walking on the street with good friends when my left leg gave out again, and I fell the very same way I had at the theater. It took five minutes to get me back up. Clearly, the pinched nerve was causing problems.

Early November, I finally contacted the neurological practice to which I had been referred a few months earlier. A week later, on a Friday afternoon, I was in the neurologist's office for more than two hours. He wouldn't look at me, but he pushed and pulled and hammered and scratched, and at the end of the appointment he said, "I want you to get a series of blood tests so that we can look for heavy metal and other types of causes. I want you to arrange for an EMG here, and after these are completed set up an appointment with me. Oh, and bring your wife."

"Bring my wife? That sounds a bit ominous."

"I find that these things go better when the spouse is present."

I now knew something was wrong. Terribly wrong. But the neurologist wouldn't tell me what he thought it might be. Clearly from his manner he suspected something, and now I would need to lay a little bit of groundwork and start sleuthing out the possible cause. I talked with Ev, trying not to project any of my concern. I talked with my boss the same way. And then I went to the Internet.

Fatigue, weakness, fasciculations: even though ALS kept coming up, I knew it couldn't possibly be ALS. More than likely, my bike riding had created an advanced case of sciatica, and I would just need to take it easy and do some physical therapy. That was my story through November, a story to hold on to until we met with the neurologist again.

2010 had all the earmarks of a good year.

The wave of positive publicity and robust sales for a book I had written about Bob Dylan's fabled Highway 61 in Minnesota carried me across the state from town to town in a book tour that had continued from the prior year. The companion documentary I had produced had its debut on public television. I was feeling accomplished and pleased that I had juggled it all, along with rising in the dark of night to do an early-morning radio news program for Minnesota Public Radio. I was unstoppable and feeling bulletproof. But there were clouds on my horizon as well.

My dad had always been an active guy with robust health, but for the past two years, our family noticed he had started to slow down. He seemed apathetic and listless. His doctor thought he was depressed, and in fact he had quietly battled depression for many years unknown to anyone except my mother. An antidepressant seemed to work for a while, but even with the medication, he would become quite angry at the smallest of slights. He would rage and growl and was especially frustrated over increasing instances of incontinence. We thought his anger was likely due to embarrassment over that very private issue. That explanation made sense.

Spring of that year also presented a new twist in my life. I was playing the supporting actress role in a personal and professional drama. My husband, a well-known radio personality, had decided to retire from his job. It was a very public decision. I was surprised by the emotions that bubbled up for me. A chapter was ending and was made bittersweet because we had met as political reporters at the Minnesota Capitol. Much of our lives together had centered on his job, even though mine was also quite demanding. I wasn't sure how our future would look.

His retirement party was May 22, 2010. I remember crying during a retrospective slide show of his career and was confused as to why. Then it hit me. I was mourning a memory of how much fun we had, how exciting and vibrant our early years had been. So much had changed. What I didn't know was how many more changes were in store for me and how important memory would become.

Two days after that party, my mother called with words that knocked the breath out of me. "Dad has Alzheimer's."

It was the one disease my father dreaded most. The news was as shocking as it was puzzling. No one in my father's family had had Alzheimer's or any form of dementia. His parents, two hard-working German immigrants, were clearheaded until the day they died. My father, who had beaten back cancer several years earlier, had said a number of times that Alzheimer's, the memory-robbing disease, was the only thing that scared him. In hindsight, it was as if he had a premonition that someday he would have to face a life without a lifetime of memories.

We arrive, check in, and sit for one, maybe two minutes. Names called, we are brought to a room unfamiliar, yet every detail remains hyperclear in my memory: floor-to-ceiling bookcases, backs bowed, shelves groaning, weighted down by the detritus of twenty-year-old neurology journals with pages torn, almost vomited from their binders, green Astroturf-like carpet, tired walls, a diploma, a certificate, attestations of qualification. He vaguely shows me where to sit, dismissing Ev to a far corner. He takes his place so that a huge, dark wooden desk separates us. He faces north, focusing his gaze on a computer screen. My chair faces south, not toward him but toward windows that never open. I have to crane my neck in order to see him. The details begin to blur. I have lost track of Ev in the vastness of this space.

It is 8:15 a.m. on December 6, 2010. Outside it is cold and dark with a northern sun just crossing the horizon. Incredibly, I find myself thinking, who reads paper journals in these times? And then he looks up, a glance that hurriedly turns back to his computer screen. The stage is set, he has placed us where he wants us—divided, conquered even before the battle, lost to each other. His only words thus far, singular syllables indicating our blocking, our places, stage right and stage left, downstage and upstage. The curtain rises.

"Well, I'll come right to the point. It is bad, as I feared. My diagnosis is that you have ALS."

The silence inside me is a bombed-out chasm, opened by the icy chill in his emotionless voice. The arrangement of the room, the barrier between us, no Ev to reach out to, no squeeze of the hand, no pat on the thigh, no human contact allowed in this most clinical of settings. I can hear the blood in my ears beating into my brain: ALS, ALS, ALS. I struggle to come back to consciousness, to find Ev in the darkness, to turn my world back the way it was where I was in control, I was the master, and I knew what I was doing. I struggle to reintroduce rational logic, thoughtful consideration, to walk around the blast site and pick up the pieces.

"I am sure that you have come to your conclusion for specific reasons," I hear myself speaking—dean of the college, calm, rational, breathing in, breathing out, chosen precisely for this moment, order into chaos. It is my first out-of-body experience.

"I am sure that you have your reasons," I say.

He walks me through quickly with no room for discussion. Blood tests: negative. EMG: indicative. Physical exam: suspicious. Upper and lower. Motor neurons. Dying. And then he offers the only warmth to be mustered in the weak sun of a Minnesota December, "There are three clinics that specialize in ALS. There are trials you can investigate." I must follow here, take notes, here is the hope. Ev is devastated, I can hear it. I can sense it. I must write this down. "There are three clinics that specialize in ALS. Where do you want me to send your records?"

Suddenly, my future is very clear. We will not be working with this man. Three clinics will soon narrow to one. Trials are not hopeful. There will be no cure. I will not get better.

We begin to shuffle, to do the things one does to signal the end of time together. But it isn't quite over.

"Often when people receive news like this, it makes them think bad things. I have to ask—do you feel suicidal?"

A response slowly composes itself, ready to be shot back in slingshot retaliation for the nuclear bomb he has just dropped on our lives: "No, but I feel homicidal." But I don't say it. I look at him, and all I say is, "No. No."

In the car, wondering if I can drive. Winter is coming, the

hoarfrost coats the few trees lining the parking lot, but the sun illuminates the next few minutes, the day yet to come, life as we know it melting in its weak light. Ev looks at me. She is crushed, bludgeoned as much by the manner of delivery as by the news.

And then she quietly says, "Couldn't they have at least given us a goddamn pamphlet?"

After peering briefly at my father's MRI scan on a computer screen, the neurologist turned to my father and said, "You have Alzheimer's. See? You see it there? That's brain atrophy. Oh yes. You have Alzheimer's."

The news left both parents stunned. My father bowed his head to his chest and sat there staring at his hands. My mother started crying. When asked what to do next, the doctor brightly suggested my father "have a good life," with the suggestion he return in six months for a checkup.

My dazed parents left with several brochures, including "Understanding Alzheimer's," which was blunt in the assessment of how much life was left. The outlook wasn't good, with five to ten years of declining mental capability, potential physical atrophy, and, finally, death.

When my mother called me with the news, all she could say, between sobs, was that he was going to forget who she was, who all of us were. How could this happen to a man who had an advanced degree, who had been an excellent teacher and a lifelong learner? A man with a quick wit and ready laugh and who was only seventy-five years old, much too young, she thought, to be walking into the deepening shadows of his life.

I had to agree with her. There wasn't a pamphlet that dealt with that kind of heartbreak.

So, there we were. A college dean and a broadcast journalist soon to meet amid the wreckage disease had flung into our separate but parallel paths.

2

THE FOOTMAN SNICKERS

I am no prophet—and here's no great matter;
I have seen the moment of my greatness flicker,
And I have seen the eternal Footman hold my coat,
*   and snicker,*
And in short, I was afraid.
    —T. S. Eliot, "The Love Song of J. Alfred Prufrock"

Unexpected, unwanted, or shocking news can sear itself into your brain. The circumstances of where and when the news was delivered: the sights, sounds, smells of whatever was happening at the time comingle with the shock and leave indelible imprints in the strangest ways.

That is why I remember the dragonflies.

After getting the phone call that my father had been diagnosed with Alzheimer's disease, I went outside to absorb the news in a forest-green rocking chair badly in need of a coat of paint that Dad and I had assembled with great difficulty some years before. I was a little surprised when a stunning pale-blue dragonfly with blue-green eyes, much too big for its body, landed on the small, round patio table next to me. The insect stood out against the cheap dark-green plastic surface with its unusual color and delicate, intricate wings. It stayed there for a while and then flew off.

Dragonflies usually appear in late summer in Minnesota, and they usually hang out around water. I was living in an urban area populated with squirrels and sparrows with not a pond, river, or stream in sight, and late spring isn't dragonfly season.

My winged friend darted back and landed on the table followed by another, nearly identical dragonfly. They both flew off only to fly back into range with several more of their kind in tow. I counted nine altogether before the entire squadron flew off. It was such an unusual occurrence that I wrote about it briefly in my journal in pages splashed with tearstains as I poured out my sadness over Dad's plight.

Months later, while reading about Native American spirituality, I learned that dragonflies are spiritual messengers, especially in the Hopi and Pueblo cultures, where the dragonfly totem is associated with change and transformation.

Those fascinating dragonflies were indeed tiny messengers. Certainly many changes were on the horizon for my family and me, and yes, some of those changes, while not pleasant, were indeed transformative.

Bruce Kramer, in the immediate weeks after his diagnosis, was also just beginning to discover how much change he and his family would have to endure, and in the early stages, Bruce, Ev, and their sons had many questions that struck at the core of their existence. How will we live? Will we be OK? These questions don't have quick or easy answers, something that our society often demands. Bruce, who has spent much of his professional career studying and practicing the concepts of good leadership, would argue that asking the questions in a different way and not accepting quick and easy answers offer far more growth and possibility. Questions with yes-no answers shut down creativity. Notice the possibilities when asking, what would it take for us to do this? which is exactly the question Bruce asked himself in the newly created shadow ALS had just cast over his life.

The sun, weak in winter's anticipation, has barely cleared the Minnesota horizon, reinforcing the darkness descending on us both. This is a crisis, a situation beyond our control, requiring the man that I am to handle it, to work it to its fruition and beyond. I am the dean of the college, and that is what deans do. Or maybe crisis is the wrong way to think about this. Be calm, breathe deeply. This is no different from another piece of music just beyond the capability of my choir. I am used to this, musicians bring form and order to the chaotic. Just follow the musical line and find the beauty before the fluttering in my gut overwhelms me, overwhelms us.

We are in the car with no pamphlet, no road map, not even a GPS to guide us. I try to project calm, to breathe deeply, but I begin to perceive a presence, overwhelming and towering over me, surrounding me, piercing me, stifling me, a doppelgänger, shadowy and demanding the full reckoning of my experience, my musicality, my leadership, my relationships, my loves, my life.

Suddenly, our future falls open like some bizarre, fantastic flower, blooming and dropping its petals around me faster than I can collect them. Even more than in the doctor's office, we see clearly that there is no solution, no grand and final ending, no heroic rise or fall. Instead, we are required to make the best from the worst, working it until it can no longer be worked, accepting with as much grace and dignity as possible an ending in the face of the pure chaos raining down into the order that just yesterday was ours. In these few hours postdiagnosis, the life we thought was ours explodes, yet the epiphany of realization remains. The phenomenon of ALS is new, but I am no virgin to its circumstance.

I have unknowingly prepared for this moment my entire life, and I am afraid.

I come from a country, a state, a county, a town, a family where for the first years of my life, projecting externally that all was well was all important. The truth was much more complex. By the time I was sixteen, tasks such as cooking and cleaning and caring for younger siblings as needed were mine. I learned to accommodate the massive breakdown of the mental illness and its accompaniments that robbed my parents of the ability, the energy to provide the internal consistency and predictability that all children require. I learned early to adapt to the changeable moods, the hospitalizations, the need to accomplish the mundane in the face of the amazing. I learned to live in chaos while all available resources focused on maintaining the ultimate outward projection—typical family, well and good.

And I learned to find solace in the specific experience of music, later in the broader call to educate and lead, but music, always music. Like a soothing balm, the times when my mother would sit at the piano, playing with heartfelt emotion and ease, brought alignment to the every-which-way existence I knew as a child. Like her father, she loved Beethoven, and I remember the strains of the Sonata Pathétique ordering our world. As I grew older and she fell away from the piano, there was still music. She loved Ramsey Lewis, Lou Rawls, George Shearing, The 5th Dimension, James Brown. And I loved them too. When she put on Ramsey Lewis, I could almost count on peace in the air. And even though I quit playing percussion in the band, mostly to register my adolescent displeasure at the noise of my existence, I still hearkened to the music that she played. When I entered high school and almost at the same time she was hospitalized, I came back to formal music training—the solace and comfort were that strong.

Music has always shown me how to order my feelings, to bring harmony into my environment, to express the inexpressible, to accomplish the impossible.

I became a teacher, first of music and then later on of education. I tried my hand at being a principal, sometimes successfully, sometimes not. As a young leader, I thought I could fix organizational cacophony, much like I fixed the chaos of my family. At first, I thought there was a single correct path in school leadership, so that in the face of complexity, I chose exclusivity, one way that oversimplified and denied the multiple points of view that invariably exist in any institution. As I look back on that time, I am afraid that I might have been disrespectful of the experience that others had, especially when they did not align with my view of how a school should operate. I made the mistakes that nearly all young leaders and too many mature leaders make: overattending to the one great goal and wishing that differences would disappear. But what I eventually gained from the experience was how to approach life with intelligence and how to work complexity with method and resolution.

And I still practiced my music, applying it to a more nuanced, pragmatic understanding of how leadership could be practiced. I began to realize a leadership aesthetic, a beauty that both hearkened back to my musical days and looked forward to a more realistic and educational way to do leadership. I stopped trying to quiet the noise that so reminded me of growing up, and I remembered the harmony that could come even when the organizational decibels were beyond the pain threshold. As a musician, I had learned to take risks without devastation, to see the face of God in the practical and technical realization of a piece, to bring whole groups of people along past the limits they thought were theirs and into a new understanding of where we might go. Through reflection and maturation, I learned to apply my musical gifts to my leadership practice.

I learned the difference between opening to possibility through questions and closing creativity with answers.

So much of leadership is about breaking down the impossible challenge into possible tasks. I learned that the impossible requires the right questions, that the right questions will frame intelligent answers, emergent and susceptible to new information rather than dull and lacking in creativity. I learned to throw myself into leadership challenges, enjoying their complexity and messiness. And even when it looked as if the problems that faced us were beyond solution, I learned to have faith that such problems were not beyond us as colleagues.

When I became dean, I knew my capabilities and my limitations, the strengths of my colleagues and the areas in which we all would need to grow. At a time in higher education when the value of theory was questioned and the cost of a professional degree was scrutinized, I found myself at deep peace with the challenge, excited to begin. I was ready to work the big ideas into the day-to-day tasks that determine whether a college is successful.

I believed that all my knowledge, my past successes and my past failures, had led me to this ultimate moment in my professional life. I loved my job. I loved my life, my wife, and family, and I was happy, even on the days that others might have described as the worst that could happen.

And now in December 2010, as we sit in the car without a pamphlet, in the bloom of our new circumstance, I struggle to connect with the competence that was once mine.

We feel the accelerating fall from the pinnacle of our life, down to the deepest trough of despair we have ever known. When we arrive at our home, we hug and we cry and hug some more, and then we retreat as if each other's presence is too much—Ev to the sunroom and I to the office. Each of us looks for some miraculous answer, knowing full well that there are no answers that can begin to approach this unbelievable turn of events. Yet, we cannot help ourselves. Perhaps this time, a hidden treatment, an unknown cure might emerge. Isn't that the power of the information age?

Ev looks up ALS and immediately stumbles upon YouTube videos about feeding tubes and ventilators. I google ALS, and my first choice is a video of Jack Kevorkian coercing an ALS patient to die. The answers are clear: there is no hope, there is no possibility, there is no value, life with ALS is over. ALS will kill us both.

In the naïveté of my knowledge of what is to come, the complexity of prioritizing our choices looms large. Questions, considerations that are singular in their approach, yielding answers that will only dull the life ahead of us, yes or no, right or wrong, burying any possibility, obfuscating any hope, are of no use to us. We must ask questions that will open new horizons. How shall we grow into the demands of what is beyond us? In the beauty of my choral art, the practicality of my leadership aesthetic, the questions I must now consider loom larger.

We cannot afford the noncreative.

The diagnosis of ALS overwhelms the life I owned just yesterday. How will I grow into the demands of that which is beyond me? What are the consequences for my Ev and our two beloved sons? Already in the first hours after the diagnosis I can see a gray pall falling over my one true love. We are best friends, lovers in every sense of the word for over thirty years. How do we conserve the precious gift of each other, the overused yet oh so true cliché that we are soul mates, when my entire physical capacity will fail? Since ALS will take my body, what will become of the spirit that has infused us so joyfully? Practical questions begin to tower over us. How can we live in a hundred-year-old up-and-down Victorian house? With projected expenses, how will we avoid becoming destitute? What are the financial implications if I cannot work? What are the emotional implications if I cannot move? What will be the consequences for Ev of caregiving? In these first hours after diagnosis, ALS feels like a death sentence as the questions carom around us, first uttered by one and then the other, back and forth and back again.

The entire experience of ALS—medically, emotionally, spiritually—seems designed to kill us.

In the first hours after diagnosis, I am terrified, but I make a decision. Fifty-four years of life experience—chaos and beauty, leadership and music—and I now know that I must bring everything I have learned to bear upon this crisis, or we will be utterly destroyed. Somehow, someway, I must turn ALS on its ear and transform it into a life sentence instead. I cannot do this alone. I will need an inner circle, family and friends and professionals, to share ideas and grief and anger. I know what I must do, but I do not know yet how I will do it.

Above all, I know I cannot fix this. That would only be childish. All I can hope is to work it, and perhaps some way forward will emerge.

3

A HOUSE BUILT ON SAND

Most of us live our lives according to an unspoken set of assumptions. We assume, for instance, that we'll make good money, live in good health, and enjoy good friends, good sex, and a good time before dealing with the endgame when it comes. Of course that is a gross simplification, but you get the idea. Many of us assume our loved ones will also enjoy robust health and well-being. I assumed my parents would live into old age in relative good health, only to die peacefully in their sleep.

We experience a rude awakening when those assumptions are turned upside down and inside out—when that happens, some of us leap into a frenzied drive to make things right, to fix the problem.

I'll admit to being a first-class fixer. Upon my father's diagnosis of Alzheimer's, later to be rediagnosed as frontotemporal dementia (FTD), I flew into fix-it mode, trolling the Internet for the latest research into the disease as well as using my medical contacts to ask questions and seek information on this perplexing form of dementia. As crazy as it sounds now, I thought that if my father's condition couldn't be fixed (and all signs clearly pointed in that direction), then maybe it could be held at bay with a battery of supplements, anti-inflammatories, exercise, and enriching activities that would preserve the remaining undamaged neurons in his brain. It became like a ragtag army's last stand to hold its position against a much stronger foreign invader. That exhausting effort probably bought a little more time, but the battle was lost on March 3, 2014, when complications of lymphoma, not dementia, felled my father.

It is easy to think that Bruce has run up against something that he can't fix. His body, ravaged by the advancing ALS, will not be healed, and he realizes that. That isn't the lesson Bruce has learned. He writes, "All of us need to find the holy balance between the fixable and the inevitable." It is knowledge hard won and a lesson many of us will learn soon enough.

> *Teach me the measure of my days,*
> *Thou maker of my mortal frame.*
> *I would survey life's brief and narrow space,*
> *and learn how frail I am.*
>
> —Isaac Watts

It is now summer in Minnesota, my fourth summer with ALS. The metamorphosis wreaked on my body, my mind, my spirit is the measure of my days, summarized in a psalm, poetized in the mind of an eighteenth-century rhymer. Remarkably, I have a record, a blog, musings, and philosophical wanderings, real-life happening, a survey if you will—both public and intimate—of the assumptions and measurements made through each small loss, slice by slice, by ALS. How easy it would be to look back one year, two years, three years and be embarrassed by the naïveté of the reflection. But grant me a little space here. I was doing the best I could, and the knowledge that continued to clarify, moving toward today's current "wisdom of the sort," was a lot like holding up a kaleidoscope where every turn showed a different pattern, each more beautiful and terrible than the last.

This is the kind of thinking that summer in Minnesota inspires.

In my fourth summer of ALS, I find it harder and harder to remember the old normal assumptions that served as a foundation for my able-bodied life. But I can remember a few. If only

I could eat correctly, exercise enough, hold all things to moderation, devote myself in equal measure to my family and my job, I would have a great chance of living past ninety and looking back on a life well lived. I remember joking that I wanted my epitaph to be "He died racing semis on his bike." There is such a human arrogance to these assumptions, and I weep in empathy for that old normal person. The assumptions were like a sand foundation on which I built my life. It took one major storm to splinter my life along the fault lines that we carry as able-bodied persons, the irrational belief that we will control how we live and how we die.

Now I move neither my arms nor my legs; I have no semblance of fending for myself; I am totally reliant on my caregivers. My rebirth, now four summers old, is a series of circles moving from loss to loss to loss until I am back to something I must lose again. The droop of the toe becomes the flop of the foot becomes the loss of the leg becomes the inability to support weight in a standing position. In so many ways, is this not the normal pathway on which all humans find themselves? Is this not a normal progression, just speeded up? The hardscrabble work of keeping up with the losses as they cascade one upon the other, finding the meaning in each drop of water flung over the edge of life's waterfall, is something I can point to from this vantage point of advanced disease as necessary to growth even as I diminish, pulled into the essence of what it means to be a living human being. I am just aging exponentially faster than most.

I know what you are thinking—that you don't need this right now, you don't want to think about it, that you have plenty of time. Tra la la, live for today, gather ye rosebuds, blah blah blah. You would be totally correct in thinking this way, until you suddenly need a way of thinking in the immediate right now that accounts for when your time has dwindled, compressing itself into what you have left. The assumptions of a long life are like the sands under our foundations, powerful and hard to resist, a natural response so that life appears to be somewhat happy—a foot-to-the-pedal, gas-powered, four-hundred-horsepower response that does not veer easily into despair.

I get this, I really do.

My spiral has been one of an able-bodied fix-and-cure mentality, circling down to the deep reflection of what it means to acknowledge loss, to finally learning acceptance and gratitude for what I have. The archetypes of my unconscious that have emerged and fallen along the way are many—white knights in shining armor and elderly women stating obvious wisdom. I have moved from unconsciously seeking the cure—the absolute rebuttal of the natural way of things—to consciously embracing the reality of frailty. This new foundation, built upon the acknowledgment of just how fleeting is life, is a foundation of stone that resists all hubris.

Isaac Watts knew the irony, and it doesn't escape me either.

> See the vain race of mortals move
> as mere shadows o'er th' eternal plain.
> They rage and strive, desire and love;
> but all the noise is vain.

December 2010, and Evelyn and I are on the phone with our dear friend Madelyn, a person we have known since we lived in Cairo, Egypt, twenty years ago. Evelyn is downstairs, and I am in our bedroom looking out on the dark street. All three of us are crying—ALS seems like such a death sentence in its early guise. While we are talking and I am looking out the window, I see people walking their dogs, the couple from across the street leaving their car and going into their house, a few kids from up the street squeezing the last bit of play out of the day, sneaking a forbidden cigarette before they have to go in to do their homework. It is all so normal, so commonplace, and I am angry, I am hurt, and I admit that I am scared that life can go on so easily. I am incredulous that the bottom has dropped out of my normal, yet normal continues. How can life proceed so matter-of-factly outside our house when my friend, my spouse, and I are in such deep grief?

And then it hits me, *this is the new normal.*

I will always carry this weird feeling, this presence as if an unwanted person stands between me and those with whom I wish to engage, this hole in the gut that will never be filled. And around me, others will behave as if all is well because they know no difference, because it is what we have learned, because if we move into the space that is left by our own disease we may not find our way back. I cannot fix this. I cannot cure it. I can only embrace the emptiness and the pain and hope that I will grow through it. This is the foundation that looks like sand but is in fact stone, and it is the surface on which I must build what is left of my life.

You can imagine how hard this is for a person who thought through the endgame and backfilled the strategies in order to get to a desired place. For example, I knew that we had to move out of our lovely up-and-down Victorian home. I knew that the reality of the stress of stairs would make it impossible for us, for me, without significant modification. So we decided to move, to prepare our home for selling, to downsize, to find a place that would accommodate what we were being told was coming in terms of physical loss but could barely imagine given our able-bodied experience up to this point. In the past, my old normal would have been to plan this, to do the lion's share of the work, to happily box up the things we would keep and sort out the things that would go. But I could not be the one who packed up and trimmed down such a household. ALS is nothing if not massively fatiguing, and I just did not have the strength. And we were beginning to realize that Evelyn could not do it on her own either. Already, the physical needs of my support had strained her elbows so that she could not lift anything with much weight. All we could do was accept the help of friends and family, turn over the intimate evidence of our lives to good-hearted people, and be grateful for the help. There would be no fix, no cure, no avoidance of this fact.

The archetype of the independent American has great strength and greater vulnerability. Disease was teaching me that independence as a foundational belief would result in catastrophe. The foundation of strong and independent living was so vulnerable to deconstruction by ALS, and the speed by which it happened was so lightning quick that to remain in such a space could only be harmful. We needed a new archetype, an unconscious avatar that mixed the dependence that was our new reality with the strength that it takes to make such change. The emergence of such a being does not come without cost.

You have to accept the fact that fixing is a lie.

Fixing is a strong temptation. To believe that I might be able to make things completely right comes honestly to me as a person who worshiped at the altars of American individualism. But for me, the demarcation between old normal and new normal is so complete and specific, so compelling, that I realized that to try to bring the old religious symbols of fixing with me into this new, ALS-defined space would only exacerbate the demise of the person I knew that I had to become. Out of the emptiness that was once the surety of my life came the question, what will you be from here into eternity? The question smacked of the apocalyptic Four Horsemen that revealed all manner of God's presence in my life. Therefore if I threw in my lot with trying to fix this, I would only be frustrated and bitter, and while I might glimpse the old normal Godhead from time to time, the person I wanted to become could not fix this.

The revelation healed me, and suddenly the foundation on which I would build whatever future might be given to me looked like sand in its vulnerability but was solid as stone in its ability to bend with the downpour of what was to come.

All of us come to realize the movement and measure of loss in each day, the crushing noise of our human vanity. And it takes every bit of energy we can muster to reach above this fog, to ask for healing when none can be found, forcing the question, how long, and how long? Read between these lines of disease, and you will recognize the spiritual strength I receive from my sons, my wife, my friends, and the human engagement for which I still have the strength. And in the end, there is the answer, the foundation measured out in dribs and drabs of energy and strength.

In my fourth summer of ALS I am healed by music and vulnerability.

There are many musical settings of Psalm 39. Admittedly, the frailty, the human vanity, the realization that we are here only for a moment and then we are gone speaks worlds to me, but just as music focuses measures of my mortality, so too does music illuminate a different meaning for the same. Johannes Brahms set Psalm 39 in his *German Requiem,* only he continued past the sadness by asking, "And now Lord, what do I wait for? My hope is in you." I guess I can admit to measures of strength from an old German agnostic's take on life's frailty.

And in the breath of those measures, I can see my way through the immeasurable, as hard as it has been and will be. You can also.

4

A DELICATE DANCE

Ever watch young children at play? It's uninhibited, spirited, and noisy, and in the process some tender feelings can get hurt as youngsters learn how to get along with one another. Kids tend to make friends easily. Adults find this task harder.

Busy schedules and lives that aren't as rooted in a single place make starting and maintaining friendships challenging. Adults are also more cautious, selective, and fearful—traits that can quickly slam the door shut on a budding friendship.

How then do two people who first warily circle each other engage in a deeper relationship? It involves intricate choreography that requires trust and honesty and one thing that scares most adults: vulnerability. It's a dance that no one should sit out.

Have you ever tried to talk about death? In some ways it is much easier with a group of strangers, people unknown except by their acquaintance through some third party, a summer gathering or winter night where well into the second bottle of wine, the topic arises. And usually in these soirées, it is treated like jazz, a topic that follows a set chart with dark sunglasses and mock turtlenecks and black shoes marking time until it is your turn to riff.

But try to talk about death with people who mean everything

to you, and the conversation is not nearly so confident. The beat increases, rhythmic anxiety and chord progressions that seem to have no clear pattern—piano, bass, and drums out of time even as the full meaning of the discussion becomes clear. To talk about death with loved ones, you must dance, leaving the jazz behind, lightly following the steps, a waltz, placing your hand in the small of the back, guiding just so, mirroring the steps—step, step, slide; one, two, three, one, two, three—synchronized, whirling with eyes on one point so that your passion leaves you breathless but not dizzy. You must embrace the topic, your beliefs, and yes, each other with whispers of silk, like lovers who must leave one another after a night's passion, not knowing exactly how to say good-bye.

It is a most delicate dance.

Disability inspires much the same. The temporarily able-bodied exhibit a wide range between comfort and discomfort when confronted by those of us who have disabilities, often reciting a litany under their breath of some variation on a theme of "There but for the grace of God, go I." And probably, if any of us stops to think carefully, we understand that God doesn't give a damn whether one of us has disabilities and another does not. The godless see it as nature's roulette, and the religious realize that what is important is what you do with your circumstance. The fact of the matter is that we are all going to die. So disability inspires its own delicate dance, one that ranges from overacknowledgment, talking very loudly and slowly to a person in a wheelchair, for example, to underappreciation—looking through the person with disability, lacking the compassion to see a heightened need for help from a fellow human traveler.

Acknowledge disability or death, and suddenly you must acknowledge just how vulnerable the human condition truly is.

It is hard to embrace the bad things that happen in life. We learn to get through them, taking a "this too shall pass" attitude, so that the idea of fully engaging the negative just doesn't surface. When discussing perceived danger, psychologists point to the animal response of fight or flight. It is a primal reaction, often ascribed to an evolutionary reptilian portion of the brain.

Thus, a person diagnosed with cancer often adopts a "fighting" lexicon. Fighting the disease is encouraged, from radiation and chemotherapies to vivid imagery therapy where the patient imagines good cells fighting and defeating cancer cells. Or sometimes people choose the flight option, denying the condition for as long as possible, until the reality cannot be denied any longer. With disease, we see denial as less than ideal. But deep down most of us understand its attraction.

What do you do when the news is bad and will only get worse? Progressive diseases, dementia, ALS, certain cancers, organs that fail, even old age—all offer no reasonable possibility that a cure can be found. Embracing the disease is the farthest thing from our minds, especially when the news is particularly bad. Most assuredly, it is not encouraged by our culture. Neither fight nor flight possesses the nuance for the complexity and inevitability of loss that cannot and will not be fixed. Instead, they suggest a vulnerability most of us find hard to face. But the human reality is that we will all face just how vulnerable we are.

Early after my diagnosis, when I could still walk but only with the support of a cane, I came face-to-face with my own denial in a pizza parlor in the Minneapolis skyway. I had tottered my way down the skyway to get a slab of the local New York–style pizza—a real slab of pizza. I ate at this place only once in a blue moon, mostly because the lines were long and also because the pieces were hugely caloric. I got into the line behind a guy in a motorized wheelchair. He ordered, got his two pieces and a bottle of Dasani, and went to the back to eat. When I struggled to the back as well, three items in two hands plus a cane, I put my stuff down—no easy task I might add—sat, and immediately realized I'd forgotten napkins. I got back up and looked over at the guy in the wheelchair, and here is the important part: so did half the restaurant. The guy had arthritic hands, there was grease from the pizza running down his arms, and he too had no napkins. How can you not see that? Just like you don't see a guy trying to balance three objects in two hands—that is how. I offered to get napkins for him, and he gratefully said, "Thanks, and do you think you could open my water for me?"

I came to call this type of interaction "The Look." We see things. We see the guy on crutches, on a cane, the woman in a wheelchair. But The Look goes right through them. We are afraid to acknowledge their disabled regalia, how they struggle, walk without balance, or don't have a free hand when one is needed. I don't mean everybody. That wouldn't be fair. I've had people hold the door for me as often as they have pushed right through it, just fast enough for the door to close in my face. Giving The Look is probably just too easy, and I must admit I know this from experience. In my old normal, I gave The Look as often as I didn't, secure and confident in my able-bodiedness. I know how good I was at The Look. I'd look right through disability, and I wouldn't have to face its possibility in the person that I'd looked through.

It is obvious that The Look is neither fight nor flight but denial in the present, a refusal to join the dance.

And there it is. It is remarkably easy to look through the reality with which each of us lives. All of us will die, and most of us will face some form of decrepitude in the process of our lives. So embracing that which brings us to death for what it can teach us—even an expanded life—is a logical thing to do. But it is hard to see that it makes sense until you absolutely must. And to look through is way too easy.

To dance this dance, we must embrace vulnerability. That isn't an easy thing to do in a society that values independence, control, and, most of all, the myth of immortality.

And this brings me to my own personal dance: whether to tell this story publicly, and whether to trust a journalist whom I have known only as a chipper early-morning voice on my radio.

A mutual friend introduced us, saying that he thought the blog I was writing for the sake of keeping friends and family informed would actually make good journalism. Cathy and I met, and we danced. I wondered if I could maintain the energy to be honest as ALS progressed. She wondered about her own journalistic integrity. In reflecting on our first meeting, she wrote:

> I wrestled with the question of whether I could cover one
> man's journey into death while keeping a journalistic arm's

length away. Could I remain a cool, detached journalist hiding behind my armor of objectivity and impartiality while fully covering Bruce's very human story? Bruce said that disease is a shared experience. He felt that talking about ALS and being honest about his experience would allow someone else to be brought into his reality if only for a moment. Being part of Bruce's experience would mean I was going to have to be fully present with him and his family. My normal journalistic detachment wasn't going to cut it.

As Cathy and I danced around each other, carefully considering whether we could trust the other to do what needed to be done—and even more so whether we might have the personal wherewithal to see this through—personal vulnerability became the theme. Again, from Cathy's journal:

> How could I saddle myself with someone's heartbreak when I was dealing with my own? I was so physically exhausted from my job as an early-morning radio host, work that demands a lot on very little sleep. Most importantly, what hit me hardest was the obvious: Bruce Kramer was going to die. Of course, we all die, but Bruce was going to meet Death sooner than most. I was being asked to invest a lot of time and energy in a project that had a very clear outcome, and I wasn't sure how I was going to tell that story. Death was the deal breaker. As I hit the garage door opener at home, I knew I didn't have the emotional strength to tell Bruce's story properly. I thought I was at peace with my decision, then as I pulled into the garage and let the door close, I surprised myself by starting to cry.

You can lose your soul when you tell this kind of story, but you can also gain a much deeper sense of your own humanity.

Vulnerable is a term we never think to apply to ourselves. It drips of a nonexistent control, of total dependency. It's the younger, more vital version of the person we think we are rearing up and crying, "Not me, not me ever!" Vulnerable is rowing a boat in unfamiliar waters—choppy and dark—uncertainty slapping at the bow. Eventually, it becomes harder to see the shore as darkness descends, our bodies exhausted from the effort.

Between the external denial from The Look and the internal realization of just how vulnerable each of us truly is, embracing our circumstance is really the only logical choice. And in the embracing is an openness that reveals the best of our humanity. When we are closed to vulnerability's gifts, we also close ourselves to living fully into the magnum opus of what is our life. I like to think of it in terms of one of my favorite pieces of music, Johann Sebastian Bach's Mass in B Minor.

It was not uncommon for composers in Bach's time to borrow heavily from earlier works they had written, or even from the works of others. What we now consider to be plagiarism, they considered to be high compliment. The Mass in B Minor is Bach's magnum opus, and in his borrowing to write this gigantic work, he borrowed from his own very best work. It was as if in turning to the final months of his own life, he looked back upon the very best that he had accomplished, integrating it into the life he chose to portray in this beautiful work. Is that not a lesson for all of us?

To be vulnerable is to examine our lives and their meaning with microscopic reflection. To be vulnerable is to take the very best that we have learned and pay it forward into the centuries to come. I admire Bach the composer, but I more admire the man who showed us a way to move forward with honesty and integrity and all of the skill and wisdom he had amassed as he completed his greatest work. You don't have to look through something or someone in denial, you don't have to dance around disability and death.

You just embrace the dance as your very own.

5

DISEASE AND DIS EASE

Webster's Dictionary is clear and succinct in its definition of *disease*: a condition that prevents the body or mind from working normally.

In the case of ALS (amyotrophic lateral sclerosis), also known as Lou Gehrig's disease, the motor neurons in the brain and spine that communicate with most of the body's voluntary muscles stop functioning normally. They die off. Communication between the tiny cells serving as a pathway from the brain to muscles is severed, and the muscles wither and decay down to the ones that, ultimately, help us breathe. It isn't known yet what causes this slow die-off of motor neurons, and there aren't any decent treatments for the disease other than one drug, which buys only a few precious months of life.

I learned all of that in a crash course on ALS in the days before I was to talk with Bruce for our first official interview about his life with the incurable disease. I knew my listeners would want to know what symptoms first set off alarms for Bruce, how far he was in a checklist of physical dysfunction, and how he and his family were handling life with the disease. I figured it would be a pretty basic first interview. It quickly turned into a much deeper conversation.

"You're blogging very eloquently about your journey on the Internet, and you're calling it Disease Diary," I began. At this point, I was gently interrupted by the affable Bruce.

"No," he corrected. "It is Dis Ease Diary. Dis. Ease." Then he smiled and waited.

I paused, wondering where this was going. "You're deliberate about using the word in that manner, Bruce. Why is that?" And so began a lesson in a concept that is powerful in its simplicity, and remarkable in its evolution. Dis ease. He explained that it goes beyond the physical, and each of us carries our own particular form of it: physical, social, cultural, personal, spiritual.

Over the years since that first meeting, Bruce has grown and refined the concept of dis ease in direct opposition to disease. One is a medical condition with the expectation of a cure, whereas dis ease is the choice we are given: whether we will live our all-too-short lives fully. Or not.

The diagnosis of disease is seductive. If you aren't prepared, if you do not strap yourself to the schooner's mast, you can shipwreck your soul on disease's sensuous song. Like a siren of aching ecstasy, blinding your perception so that your intellect, emotion, desire cleave sensuously to your new lover, disease drowns you in its sensations. Light diffuses, vision blurs, sound muffles, and your very breath feels as though it will explode, holding you under in murky depths. Disease seduces you into thinking it is all about you, your diagnosis, your condition, your treatment. You can be seduced by images of fighting and battles and metaphors of winning and losing. Disease tricks you into believing a cure is the only healing story. And then, disease grasps you and dashes you against rocks that will not yield, beating you into splinters of self-absorption until the person you were is no longer recognizable, until the seduction is complete, and it is too late.

I remember the seduction like a first lover's face.

December 2010, and I am reborn in diagnosis, without sextant or stars or maps to guide me. The neurologist's words ending with the mantra, "ALS, ALS, ALS." It is as if he has tossed me overboard into roiling seas. I search for any way to stay afloat, to come up for breath. His voice, urging me into uncharted waters where disease lies now exposed and the danger is beyond comprehension, and he ironically introduces me to self-harm with a question in the guise of care. "Do you feel suicidal?"

Suddenly, I am sailing a different ship with a different crew, too close to the rocks where sirens sing, "There is no cure, only disease; there is no cure, only death." This is not the ship I boarded, this is not the odyssey I joined in some youthful indiscretion, the excitement of going to war boiling a young man's blood, nor the fictional account of some other plunging into the deep abyss of epic adventure.

Suddenly, I realize that I am no Odysseus.

I consider my new peers, PALS: People with ALS. Hopelessly afflicted, welcomed into a sisterhood, a brotherhood defined by constant and steady physical loss. The realization slowly emerges that some of us will never understand what brought us here. Some of us will never recover from the diagnosis of disease. Some of us are already on the rocks, thoroughly and utterly hopeless and starving for some semblance of the old ways we knew before—the ropes and buoys and floats and rafts that surround us offer no way back and a certain fate ahead. And some of us have learned a new way, my peers, PALS hopelessly afflicted, hopefully welcoming.

And somehow, in spite of disease, self-absorption, seduction, the temptation to do battle; somehow, in spite of senses discombobulated by the murky waters of disease; somehow, in spite of the typhoon diagnosis, crystal clear in its meaning; somehow, in spite of the violence of the birth—somehow we are reborn into a new life christened by ALS.

Six days later, I begin to write. In the writing comes clarity, a way forward, a nagging, gut-gnawing hunch that this singular story line of a progressive neuromuscular disease is the flinty grit of a most human narrative. As I write, the advent of diagnosis fades into my first epiphany: that an ALS-only story will restrict me, cinch itself around my intellect and emotions and spirit, squeeze out any possibility of exploration and growth in favor of campfire tales with ghosts of bodily breakdown, the things I cannot do, the horrors of utter physical failure lying ahead. The more I consider the implications and inferences of ALS, the more I come to understand disease's seduction, how it will limit my life to a minuscule portion of what it might be in the massive unknown yaw of time that remains. Sixty days later, in spite of disease, it becomes clear to me, and a chronicle—broader, more human, more honest, more indicative of what I know could be— slowly emerges. I begin to write my dis ease—a public journal, a blog, a diary of dis ease—though I cannot yet see beyond its emergence.

I considered the word *disease*, its etymology a plaything, a toy to be tossed back and forth and explored, a bit of tongue-in-cheek, a bit of truth. Split it, divide it, dissect and analyze and recognize. And in that recognition, the concept exploded—dis ease. In the beginning, dis ease was what I glibly and too nonchalantly described as "dissing the ease," but over time its meaning grew, taking me into new terra firma, new definitions of being alive.

Slowly the realization dawned.

Dis ease had always been with me, lying in depths of collective human need, illuminating life's inevitable sharp edges, its dangerous borders, its precarious balance between good living and catastrophic existence. Now I could see it. Dis ease is true love, soaring in the stratosphere, yet plummeting to earth in betrayal unforeseen. Dis ease is the newborn child, perfect in every detail, vandalized by the reality of overwhelming disability. Dis ease is loyalty to a career path, a good job, a life goal realized, taking a different turn and becoming wholly untenable. Dis ease is the good life interrupted by the pain and suffering of those we love, the diagnosis or sudden news plunging lives into despair, scrabbling for some hope of a good life yet to be. There is not a person who does not know dis ease, boiling the pit of their gut, on the tip of their tongue, in their muscle memory, in the discord between the life they know and the life they fear.

Slowly the realization dawned: We are all dis eased.

As I began to comprehend the meaning of dis ease, the meaning of ALS, I could see the physical breakdown looming on my horizon, but dis ease revealed so much more. Hard to pin down, hard to define, dis ease emerged as an ever-evolving framework that went where I went, did what I did, was as I was, always in the room like oxygen or fire, and not just for me but for everyone. I came to know how restricting calamity to its essential manifestation, whether ALS or cancer or heart disease or schizophrenia or autism or any other of the myriad physical and emotional maladies that visit themselves on humanity, was ludicrous.

I learned quickly the collective nature of dis ease. In the sharing of my ALS diagnosis, a moment of ALS truth emerged. Friends and family and colleagues constructed with me a quiet yet troubled space, a realization of their own variations on my ALS theme: "I have cancer." "I am sick with depression." "My husband doesn't love me anymore." "The pain in my legs is unbearable." I realized their story lines were awakenings, profound connections in the moment of shared revelation that each of us carries uneasiness, often unacknowledged but always present; that each of us, as we come in contact with the reality of mortal disease, has to process what this new reality means. It upset the certainty in the lives of my friends and family and colleagues, just as it established new certainty in mine.

My diagnosis revealed the rocky shores beneath our lives, and disease tempted self-centeredness. Our dis ease, shared between us in intertwining threads of ALS and cancer and depression and hurt and pain, was the greatest revelation of all.

Not everyone is open to such truth. Not everyone wishes to strip off the incapacity that dis ease exposes. We are taught that dis ease is easily managed by the right life, the right beliefs, the right partners, the right jobs, the right nationality, the right possessions, the right dreams. We are told that dis ease is easily held at bay. Avoid disease, and the dis ease spawned by the very act of living does not have to exist. Until we experience disease, we don't know how bounded, how delimited, how inadequate are our abilities. The sudden reality of ALS was like a dreary, sad, and fearful lake of standing water, waiting to be plowed and splashed upon everyone who mattered. Dis ease acknowledged the reality but also opened us—me, my wife, my kids, my family, my friends, my colleagues—to hope and even possibilities of joy.

Disease takes you to the precipice of horror. Dis ease offers beautiful vistas of hurt and healing and hope.

I have experienced joy and hope where sorrow leads to collective laughter, collective horror leads to strength in numbers, and known endings open new beginnings. My physical condition will never be cured, but dis ease allows me to be healed by the presence of those I love, to perceive aliveness that I never perceived, to recognize that joy and sorrow are from the same source, and that living fully is energy created from catastrophe and hope. I have learned that physical loss is metaphysical, that holy Spirit is in breath suppressed, and that those sources that give me the greatest joy can cut me to the quick while lifting me beyond any happiness I might have known.

There is disease and dis ease. Disease is loss by design, with whole industries devoted to cures as if such a thing were possible. Dis ease gives us choice. We can awaken and pay attention to the entire narrative, or we can deny and pretend unawareness. We can be seduced by the siren song, or we can lash ourselves to the mast and hold on for dear life. No matter the choice we make, dis ease remains—my informant, my teacher, my mentor, my constant companion.

And my awakening is a masthead from which I will live and die.

6

FAITH, PART I

Fulfilling What Is Meant to Be

In October 2012, Bruce quit working. For the first time in forty-five years he didn't get dressed and head out the door for another day of work. He had continued to shoulder the heavy responsibilities of leading the College of Education, Leadership, and Counseling at the University of St. Thomas after being diagnosed, preferring to continue to work on behalf of budding educators rather than give in to the growing demands of ALS. But after twenty-two months, the disease had sapped his strength to the point where he needed to step aside. As was his custom, Dean Kramer carefully crafted a succession plan and outlined his exit strategy, executing it as best he could.

During one of our recorded conversations for radio, I asked him how he would think of himself once he stopped working. Many people make the mistake of blurring their lives with making a living. Bruce answered thoughtfully that perhaps influenced by his musical background (where musicians think of themselves as musicians first, then what they do and where they do it and for whom), he would continue to think of himself first and foremost as a teacher.

I guess I'll always consider myself a journalist, even after I leave the daily grind of the newsroom. Part of my job is ferreting out the truth as much as possible, and by working with Bruce, I've had to come to grips with one of life's great truths. Bodies break down. They are designed to do just that. Medical science can prop up our mortal containers only so long before they simply give out. We would all be better served if we accepted the inevitability of physical loss because it is barreling down on us like a coal train out of Montana. Trying to leap off the tracks isn't going to save us.

Bruce feels great spiritual fulfillment in recognizing what is meant to be and accepting the losses, but such knowledge doesn't come easy.

Saturday morning, misty gray. Foggy, cold dewdrops hang from branches of trees recently colored and now deep brown and black and sad. I cannot say that I am unaffected by the scene framed by my window. Somehow, the picture outside mirrors the me inside, working through another chapter in the diary of my circling back home, too reflective of the fog and damp, too conscious of the new life lessons dis ease continues to thrust upon me—this educational guest I did not invite to visit with me or anyone else I love. If I can just part the curtain of noise and haze, clear the fog off the path, carefully choose the toeholds and fingerholds down to the quiet center, a small ember, a tiny light burning, telling me to be still and know, I will again have faith and belief that this is nothing.

In the book of Job in the Common English Bible, God asks, "Where were you when I laid the earth's foundations?"

What could be so hidden, so misty, so obscured? A new song emerges, and I must learn to sing it. Arrhythmic, with unfamiliar tempo, strange melodies, atonal harmonies where engagement and work and institution no longer exist in tonal consonance. The sense of purpose that I knew as a teacher, professor, dean is now just memory. It is a place where demons tread, mocking questions in the night, purposeless rolling around the condo by day—what good are you now if you do not work? No response can adequately answer, and it never could. Consider it honest documentation of the path, for the question arises no matter what—I was inculcated, powerfully reinforced to tie work and self together in an intimacy reserved for lovers. And while I saw it coming—the day when I left, when I gave up the responsibilities, the day when I achieved the ultimate enlightenment of loss—the leaving still remains. And I rattle around the modern prophet's question, "What good am I?"

God asks, "Who is this darkening counsel with words lacking knowledge?"

It's not that I won't get through this, that I don't see the necessity and the rightness of what I have done, that my worth suddenly plunged off a cliff once I stopped working. But my heart's emotion is still catching up with my head's logic. Feeling is the hare in the race—fast out of the gate, yet falling behind the tortoise of well-worked thinking. And both sides of me, the feeling and sensing, the thinking and analyzing, intertwine back and forth, a roadway of rollers where speed and momentum get you through only the first climb of quasi-despair. Logic and sadness dictate the realization that even had I not left, had I not honored the insistent teaching of ALS, I would be questioning as I am questioning now. These are my gray fog mists, my dewdrops waiting to fall from melancholy trees to be sucked up into the dry air, evaporated before they reach bottom. And if I am honest, there is clarity in the reality, that twenty-two months postdiagnosis was a good run but would never be enough.

God demands, "Prepare yourself like a man; I will interrogate you, and you will respond to me. Would you question my justice, deem me guilty so you can be innocent?"

This week I spoke with my dear sister five time zones away, sharing the intimacy of losses both experienced and expected. She anticipates: a parent in her ninth decade, ancient and susceptible, vulnerable and old. There is nothing to say except to love the fact that such hurt is present, even though the fear is in the future moment. I have experienced such anticipation, and even for the most centered and mindful soul, such reality overwhelms the stillness. It is like biting one's tongue, only to return to the point of swelling as susceptible to another and another bite. And as we center on the anticipation and the memory and the rebirth that is still taking place, the clarifying realization emerges that it is not an easy center, and your own consciousness does not spare you from grieving and loss and hurt.

God asks, "Have death's gates been revealed to you; can you see the gates of deep darkness? Have you surveyed earth's expanses? Tell me if you know everything about it."

This week I bribed my kids to take me to the Led Zeppelin *Celebration Day* movie event. It was a full house, it was fun, and most of all it was time away from the sorrow. We bathed in waterfalls of sound washing over us, piquing us not through the profound and new but through the shared experience of rock and roll and rhythm and blues and love of my kids. I did not anticipate the lightness; I expected to be tired and a little out of sorts given the late hour. But now, in the mist and grayness of a Saturday cadence, a rhythmically struggling search for the new path, this brief time together is a memory of strength and light and smiles and joy. And Jimmy Page can still put out in a way that leaves you breathless.

God asks, "Where's the road to the place where light dwells; darkness, where's it located?"

And then there was Friday's visit by my colleague and friend and secret school principal ally, who came to see me ostensibly to talk through a couple of program opportunities back in the trenches. He showed me some of the testimonials he has collected to interpret the meaning of the work we used to do together, which he still carries on. By the end of his visit, my heart was lighter as the wellspring of twenty-five years of accrued experience was tapped and opened, relieving the pressure that self-worth's questions can build. Did he really come for a consultation, or did he just sense that for a friend such a conversation would offer the briefest of needed respite from the circling down to the inevitable? I don't know, and I doubt if he would say, but I know that the discussion was good for my soul, and it allowed me to plunge back into the necessary darkness of working this out.

Job answers, "Look, I'm of little worth. What can I answer you? I'll put my hand over my mouth. I have spoken once, I won't answer; twice, I won't do it again."

I'd like to pretend that there was some large message, some portent of a greater awareness, a higher consciousness, a communion with God that I could point to over the past week. But I have experienced nothing so large or significant. It has been mist and gray and damp and cold and dewdrops waiting to fall. It has been the "dangling conversation . . . verses out of rhythm, couplets out of rhyme." It has been enforced presence, well beyond the center that I hang on to for now. And yes, for the first time in a long time, it was tears beyond the catch in the throat and the leak out the side. It was sobbing, hiccuping, snotty-nosed, cannot-catch-your-breath sorrow.

Job continues, "You said, 'Who is this darkening counsel without knowledge?' I have indeed spoken about things I didn't understand, wonders beyond my comprehension."

As I finish this writing, today is a new day, offering the best reason to live in Minnesota. Saturday's freezing rain has given way to a day that is cool and crisp and blue and sun; it lifts the spirits beyond the sorrow. I don't know how much longer I will live. I know that I am dying. But this is not new knowledge, and it is not ALS. It has always been so. Disease only changes the circumstance and the speed, but the knowledge remains as it was. The autumn sky removes the blinders, so that even sadness has a hidden joy.

Job ends: "You said, 'Listen and I will speak; I will question you and you will inform me.' My ears had heard about you, but now my eyes have seen you. Therefore, I relent and find comfort on dust and ashes."

And a still voice within continues to sing a new song.

7

THE TELL

I make my living talking about all manner of things, so I am no stranger to bad news. My career is based on it. Each day, I bring to my listeners a smorgasbord of difficult, disturbing, sometimes even horrifying stories of death and destruction, catastrophe, and cruelty. It is my job to calmly relate the news, the good and the not so good. I have done this for so long that I've developed a journalist's callus: the attitude that bad things happen, and I will matter-of-factly tell you about them. It has to be something pretty big to shake me. My father's diagnosis of FTD shook me, blasting right through me, straight to my heart—so much so that I initially allowed the idea of his dementia to muzzle me, much as dementia would ultimately muzzle my father.

Very few people outside of my immediate family knew about my father's diagnosis, and we wanted to keep it that way. Despite his stoicism, my father knew what was going on. I can't imagine how hard it was for him, the awareness that his brain was malfunctioning. Each time the word *dementia* was mentioned, my father would hang his head, as if in shame, or maybe he felt defeat. More than the cancer that he had beaten back a number of years earlier, dementia was the one disease he feared. My father had good reason to dread dementia. As with ALS, there are pitifully few effective treatments, and the outcome is almost always the same: an agonizing slide into a mental abyss where, if the disease continues, even the most basic behaviors can be forgotten.

I didn't talk about my father's dementia until, after a major fall, he wound up in a hospital and ultimately a nursing home. Once our family was engaged with these institutions, I began to notice how demeaning doctors, nurses, and aides could be, not just to him but to other patients who shared a similar fate. My father's caregivers appeared to be people who—however well meaning—were either uncomfortable, impatient, or too busy to properly interact with a person who had a failing memory. Those observations made me furious and very protective.

To advocate for my father, for the man I knew him to be, I knew that I would need to lose my reticence, the muzzle that stopped me from speaking the horrible news about my father. Instead of never speaking the name *dementia,* I began to carefully include it in conversation about my dad. And rather than focusing on the inevitable losses that I knew he would experience, I consciously decided to concentrate on what he could still do.

Without naming it, I was experiencing Bruce's observations about telling.

I discovered that when I talked about dementia, some people would knowingly nod and whisper they understood, or they would tell me their own heart-wrenching stories of a loved one's descent into a twilight world of confusion, anxiety, and frustration. Others would stare blankly, murmur some brief condolence, and walk away, clearly not interested or able to hear about something so depressing as losing one's mind.

It is revealing how people react to bad news, how we tell others about our pain, our fear, and our losses. Bruce and Ev recognized that how they revealed their life-changing news, in the process they came to call "The Tell," often uncovered the pain and dis ease carried by others, an almost archaeological revelation of pure humanness.

With the diagnosis of ALS, Ev and I realized that our new status would be both comforting and overwhelming to our friends, family, and colleagues. We knew we had to share our news, and in that knowledge, we kind of stumbled into a space that I came to call "The Tell." The Tell was both playful and spontaneous, sometimes because we set it up so that close friends could share intimately, and other times because it just happened. That experience continues today, for even though everyone close to me is aware of my ALS, its progression means that both of us still have circles that are unaware of our latest version defining yet another new normal.

The process of The Tell first came about as I would run into people who saw me with a cane and asked, "What did you do?" Invariably, my first statement was, "I didn't do anything," but I was left with the decision of The Tell—knowing how odd the person would feel if I went on to reveal why I was on a cane, and knowing how odd I would feel if I just left it up in the air.

It took me a while to figure out how to write about The Tell, partly because it was so seminal to my dis ease experience, and partly because I was afraid that I wouldn't do it the justice it deserves. *Tell* is a distinctive word. As English speakers we usually associate it with its narrative definition. This verb form is certainly key to what I'm writing about, but *tell* also has an archaeological definition that offers insights into the word. In the Middle East, a tell is a mound containing layers of civilization, one built over the other. The noun illuminates the dis ease experience, as each of us grows to become layer upon layer of events and knowledge, unease and dis ease, and comfort and joy built one upon the other. Our private archaeology mixes relics with relics, up and down the strata of our psyches. It is what makes us so complex and unique, so beautiful and dangerous.

So Ev and I constructed our own version of The Tell. At first, I think we expected The Tell to be about our own grief and shock, and to a point it was. But what I soon realized was that news like "I have been diagnosed with ALS" spawns an incredible range of reactions, and the dis ease experience is not just in the teller but also in the told. I learned quickly that there was no comfort and great comfort in telling. I learned that the profound sense of truth that I owned in my diagnosis had no bearing on the ways that friends and family reacted. Some responded with denial, others with anger. Some expressed hope, and others quiet acceptance. The presentation of our vulnerability and dis ease inspired human expression that ranged from the holy to the profane. As we shared our dis ease, we became conscious of how many of our friends, family, and colleagues carried their own dis ease as well.

This is where the archaeology of The Tell comes in, for it seems to me that each of us is like those Middle Eastern mounds: once you dig past the top layer, long buried and hidden life artifacts become apparent. Some of those artifacts are pure joy, and some are horrifying. What we learned to expect was that sharing our dis ease invited others to share theirs. Since my diagnosis, I have heard stories of terminal illness, broken relationships, physical and psychological assault, hopeless addiction, flat-out discrimination, physical challenge, abuse—dis ease that represented life loss and life hope dashed or realized. There have been many dis ease storytellers. Some would qualify their experiences—"I know that this doesn't measure up to ALS"—while others would tell me stories that made my dis ease feel like I had dodged an atomic bomb. I always understood that we humans carry our past, present, and future pains and joys, hopes and fears just underneath the veneer that we present to the outside world. I just didn't realize how present those pains and joys were. Truly, it has been like traversing an archaeological dig, with each Tell a personal story illuminating the human condition. It has been a gift of privilege and healing.

There exist institutions specific to different kinds of dis ease that help people to tell—Alcoholics Anonymous, for example. I have discovered my own institutions through the Internet forums built for my brothers and sisters in ALS. These places are raw, and yet they heal. They often predict the course of disease, but they also offer ableness in the face of breakdown. In these places, The Tell is not abstract but achingly human. Often, I see inspiration and despair in the same sentence, uttered by voices already taken. And here is one of the things that is profoundly touching: those who find a way back from the normal brink of sadness and grief invariably talk about a friend, a partner, a lover, a family, a colleague who continues to embrace them in spite of their emotional or physical condition. Those who spiral into despair believe they are alone.

I am strengthened for my dis ease by the human experience of connection. When I am able to be with those who balance their ease and dis ease so that life goes on, who reject the disabilities that others with less creativity imagine for them, and who embrace the new abilities that they have learned along the way, these people strengthen and energize me. When I imagine myself cut off and alone, my vision is literally repressed into a gray despair. I don't want to oversimplify, but when others share the new abilities they have learned from dis ease, even when these are most subtle or even unconscious, my own burdens seem less disabling and my vision seems clear.

Dis ease gives us the choice of The Tell. As a noun, it is acknowledging the messy jumble of all the layers of our experience. As a verb, it is the truthful sharing of how we feel. When I see the inevitable spiral toward the great gift that dis ease brings, I know it is the gift for which I have prepared my whole life—fully and humanly shared. Whether we wish to admit it or not—liberal or conservative, rich or poor, religious or atheist, gay or straight, black or white, English or Spanish—each one of us carries dis ease and the choice of The Tell.

To paraphrase George Burns, dis ease is not for sissies. Dis ease offers The Tell as the very human gift that can mean growth in capacity, even as ability shrinks. Through The Tell, I have learned just how resilient and brittle humans can be. Through The Tell I have seen how dis ease debilitates some and strengthens others, enhancing vision or blinding the bearer, marking where we were and indicating where we are going. It is truth in the narrative, and it is truth in the archaeology.

All of us carry dis ease. All of us seek to ease the hurt. All of us have choices, and all of us have no choice. It is the knife edge of the present that each of us walks. It is the omnipresent question: will we be strengthened by awareness of our dis eased life, or will the awareness overwhelm us?

For each of us, only time will tell.

8

IT ISN'T JUST ABOUT YOU

Given demographics and statistics, if you are not a caregiver to an ill or disabled loved one right now, odds are good you will be. As the population ages and greater numbers of people develop chronic illnesses, more health care is happening at home with relatives and friends stepping up to help. Caregiving isn't a role many of us choose: it seems to choose us. Once immersed in the experience, we find—very quickly—that nothing is easy about caregiving and that it will only get harder. It is physically taxing, time consuming, emotionally draining, and ultimately life changing.

An Internet search using the word *caregiving* reveals 2.6 million results and many very good websites that offer a wealth of information and advice. But even armed with all that knowledge, no one can be prepared to watch how disease slowly sucks the life out of a loved one. It is difficult to witness the physical losses, and if the one suffering is racked by waves of bodily pain, the sense of helplessness can be overwhelming. The anguish isn't diminished but takes on a different hue when watching a loved one struggle in the grips of addiction or mental illness. For me, most heartbreaking is to see cognitive changes unfold as personality shifts, radically changes, or worse: the loved one forgets who you are.

The lengthy and bewildering process of doctor visits, tests, hospital stays, and mountains of paperwork can be overwhelming for the patient and caregiver. What can also overwhelm is a pervasive melancholy that is difficult to shrug off, even as great effort is made to be upbeat. It isn't obvious at first, but that sadness is the mourning of all that was and dreams of what was to come. Depression is not uncommon among caregivers. It all can seem so hopeless.

Anxiety can shadow caregivers, too. Just when there is a respite or remission and the situation looks a bit brighter, or the "new normal" of disease becomes familiar and it feels safe to relax, the ground moves again, and the balance is upset.

There was a point in my father's life when the mental and physical changes wrought by dementia were layered and intertwined with ailments that surprised us when finally discovered: a full-blown, deeply entrenched bladder infection, an almost completely blocked major heart artery, a spleen ballooned to double its normal size by an insidious, slow-growing, and ultimately lethal lymphoma. Each physical symptom would pop up, and doctors would try hard to mitigate the underlying problem before another would appear. It felt like a crazy game of medical whack-a-mole. Finding stable footing was very hard when the sands of disease kept shifting. The uncertainty added to the anxiety, and in turn each fed off the other. Disease does not allow you to fully relax. There is always the fear of another tremor underfoot and the question of when.

Despite the crush of responsibilities and stress, caregiving can also be deeply fulfilling. This loving, selfless act underscores the beauty of intimate human interaction. Would that society better recognize the importance of such a powerful role and acknowledge its importance. Blessed are the caregivers!

In our fourth summer of ALS, we need to make a decision. Will my beloved go back to work in the fall? Or will she stay home in anticipation of my increasing weakness, using up every iota of her accrued leave, gambling that my time is nigh? For any family, such a decision requires a great deal of thought. We will take an enormous financial hit, paying retirement and medical insurance, while losing nearly half of our salary. At least this seems the logical way to frame the decision. Not so clear for either one of us is the psychological toll. Most certainly there will be an emotional cost, a spiritual fog she will experience if she does not have some creative outlet for the teaching that she loves, the children to whom she is so committed, the soul-felt music that emerges as the children discover that to be human is to be musical. If we can find just the right balance, this work will strengthen my one true love. And she will be more than ready for the demands of caregiving that are to come. After four summers of ALS, I have learned that caring for my beloved is the most important caregiving consideration, and for good reason.

When I was told that I had ALS, I was devastated, and not being given a lot of information by the diagnosing neurologist, I naturally turned to the Internet to discern what was going to happen to me. There is a great deal of information (and misinformation) about the progression of ALS on the Web. During those first few weeks postdiagnosis, each new revelation about ALS was hard, raw, and terrifying. And I thought it was all about me. Of course I came to this me-first perspective honestly. We are taught that tragedy is about our own reaction to it. But from all the YouTube videos, the websites, the pictures, the personal stories about ALS, something emerged for me that heightened my fear. Slowly I became aware that my ALS wasn't restricted to my experience of the disease.

The next shock for me was the realization that when we face dis ease, we face it not alone, even though we might feel that way. We face it in tandem with others, and those others suffer just as much, if not more, in the dis ease process.

I've been truly lucky in my life. When Ev and I got married, we vowed to each other "for better or for worse." I know that, at least in our country, nearly every couple makes this commitment. We usually take it further, clarifying "in sickness and in health." After my diagnosis, I found myself hovering over my memory of our marriage vows like an out-of-body experience. I remember actually looking down at these two earnest young people, Ev and me, so in love, so naive. I couldn't help it. I actually wondered, if Ev had had any inkling of what was to come, would she have cast her lot with me? On one level, it really isn't fair to ask such a thing, but on another, it is entirely reasonable, for such is the kind of thinking that comes in the traumatic aftermath of disease's diagnosis. And as I floated between memory and presence and fear of what ALS was doing to me, a persistent realization emerged: ALS care would hurt my beloved partner and my wonderful sons even more than ALS would harm me.

This was no idle fear. Research on the effects of chronic and devastating disease on people and their caregivers shows that while patients can generally reach a certain level of acceptance with a reasonable emotional response, the same cannot be said for caregivers. In other words, persons with ALS, people with Alzheimer's, diabetes, cancer, heart disease, or other diseases can find satisfaction in their lives in spite of their condition. But the same research shows a very different picture for their friends, families, and lovers. Those responsible for the care of the chronically ill are far more susceptible to despair, and their emotional quality of life can actually diminish over time. We shouldn't be surprised. The responsibilities can be crushing, and the redefinition of roles can put enormous pressure on caregivers. This is not to minimize the effects of the disease on the afflicted. I have corresponded with too many persons with ALS at the end of their emotional rope to minimize such effect. But disease has the subtlety of an atomic bomb. It smashes indiscriminately, befouling everyone within the familial and friendly circle.

We have experienced this phenomenon not only with my own family but also specifically with the adult children of people with dementia. The pain and confusion of redefining a relationship with one's parent are difficult. The realization that your mom or dad is no longer that person who took care of you, who was there for you as your greatest critic and fan, and who instead now needs the kind of care that you always associated with young children—this realization comes hard. And with dementia, often the tipping point where care needs to be heightened and roles redefined is hidden until after the moment it is needed. Logistics, finances, emotion, and confusion about the changing roles of caregiver and mom or dad or partner or spouse come together in a perfect storm of emotion and stress. Dementia strikes, and everyone in its vicinity gets dementia all over them. It is the same with other chronic diseases.

When I hear politicians and policy wonks complain about the cost of disease management, I feel like they are talking about Martians. They seem to believe that we can blame those who are ill for the repercussions of chronic disease. They bemoan the dollar costs, while pretending that the rest of humanity will never be disease afflicted. It isn't logical. Given the experience of aging, chronic disease is in everyone's future. If it doesn't affect you as an affliction, the chances are very good that it will affect you as a caregiver. We rarely think of how systemic are disease's demands. Instead, we act as if chronic disease happens to "those people," others who are on the margins of our own existence. At least, and I am sorry for this, that is how I perceived chronic disease pre-ALS, as if control could be effected and responsibility could be pinned upon the afflicted.

After four summers of ALS, such arrogance has fallen away like the scaly skin of a molting snake.

I now realize that the real issue is how to make disease management normal—normal for a society, and normal for a family. An entire side to disease management is missed, because once disease is known, it takes on a presence, almost like another person in the room. It worms its way into the intimacy of your relationships. It spins in your gut and disrupts your sense of peace. It seeks no less than total domination, if not of the conversation, then of the light and color in the spaces of your love. The balance disease demands between overwhelming consciousness and total denial would be difficult for the strongest and healthiest among us. The fact is that the real costs of disease management come in ways that are almost too difficult to measure and yet remarkably easy to perceive. Such issues do not lend themselves well to policy debate.

Our family is a case in point. As my own physical regression progressed, I became hypersensitized to how Ev picked up more and more of the daily responsibilities—laundry, food preparation, cleaning, and of course, all while she was working a full-time job. When we had not even hit the point when I needed constant care, where every small item of daily grooming would require the support of someone else if it was to be accomplished, I could mark the physical toll the responsibility was taking. And it would have been so easy to ignore it. The stress and demand that ALS made on her far exceeded the emotional and physical resources that any normal person might hope to possess.

Listen, I have seen the grimness that creeps in to the face of a caregiver. While I could gauge my own response, I had to learn the signs, the facial cues, the body language indicative of caregiver overload. And only in learning could the circle of care be completed. No person can give without receiving, and receiving will never be authentic without learning to give. And of course, the care cycle becomes more complicated as the symptoms of disease progress. I possessed less and less physical ability to mitigate the downward spiral that my increasing care required. What is to be done when you can no longer physically reciprocate care?

As we look back on the early days of my ALS care, it is hard not to be just a little embarrassed by how we muddled through, allowing each other to step up to the brink and face alone the overwhelming, larger-than-life requirements that ALS threw at us. It wasn't until our second year after diagnosis that we came to know the real toll that chronic disease management exacts. It required that we learn skills, tricks, mind-body centering in its management. We learned to pay ourselves, to conserve energy, to sit quietly and just be. All of this we had to learn in the chaos of defining what it meant to care, where chronic disease became a moving target and its demands increased daily. We came to know both the joy and the grief in the fact that the present moment was the best we could expect as ALS inexorably moved forward. And only in this learning were we able to give ourselves a fighting chance to win the wrestling match that holds despair at bay, creating the space where we would still be best friends and lovers.

And do not think that we deny that relief will come, unwanted yet highly desirable when finally attained.

Strength is only available through care, care for one's self, and care for others. Even the healthiest among us needs respite.

For the caregivers of the chronically diseased, it is the posttrauma that means the most, and respite and care are exponentially required. Over time, we learned to communicate better, to see what the other could not see, and to offer caring awareness in place of physical cure. Now, in our fourth summer of ALS, it is still more difficult than anything we have ever imagined, but the cycle of care—to give and to receive and to give again—strengthens us.

The fact is that none of us is truly finished until the great lessons have been learned. Disease has brought me this spherical lesson over and over and over again—that care for requires care of, that caregiving requires caretaking, that caring space is not only physical but deliciously, consciously spiritual. In our care for each other, I have faith that we will move through and become even more the persons we want to be, the persons we need to be. The gyre widens and spirals down into a caring that to fulfill itself must become almost transcendent.

The care for each other that we have been required to learn is now too much for it ever to be allowed to end, except in the ultimate care that is still to come.

Can you imagine such execution if it had been in the dead of winter with Ev responsible for a room full of kindergartners?

It soon became clear that the elevator would not be fixed this day. And as we began to plan for the move into a hotel (I won't even describe the logistical planning and the amount of equipment in addition to the Hoyer lift required), an idea from one of the caregivers online came through. "Have you considered calling the fire department?"

As we talked, it became more and more evident that getting me into the condo, even if I could not have my power chair, was most desirable. So Ev called the fire department. She told them, "I don't think this is an emergency, but I have no way to get my husband up to the third floor where our condo is. Is there any way you could help me?" The dispatcher on the other end stated, "I don't know, sounds like an emergency to me." And within twenty minutes three fire persons—Garrett, Lisa, and Boomer—had figured out how to slip a cloth stretcher underneath me in order to carry me up three flights of stairs. Our lovely neighbors down the hall loaned me their power chair for the next twenty-four hours.

And some off-balance balance was achieved.

This took place on a Wednesday, and I have to admit that it wasn't until the following Saturday that I began to feel like my old self again. The ALS person I have become is so easy to disrupt, so easy to push off balance, so easy to move into painful and difficult spaces, that I hardly recognize him. Yet I know it is me. I know that the energy I expend to create a space that is calm and fulfilling and centered is much more than I realize. The experience of being carried up three flights of stairs speaks of how simply the center can be pushed to the side.

I don't tell you this for sympathy or pity. I tell you this because as cliché as it may sound, disease has taught me that change is the one constant on which I can depend. And what I must continually relearn is how in the face of such constant change and loss, the gifts of joy and life emerge. I know that they do. Many times, even in my ALS normal, I've experienced joy in the face of sorrow, gain in the face of loss, constancy in the face of disruption. And yet, I have also experienced just how human and flawed I am. I continually ask myself: When will I learn that none of this is anything more than the illusion of safety? When will I learn that joy and sorrow, loss and gain, constancy and disruption are nothing more than different sides of the same human experience? When will I learn that balance requires that both the positive and negative must be present?

Sometimes, it takes the overwhelmingly physical teaching of the local fire department to remind you that the gift of spiritual space is the counterbalance of physical loss. Sometimes, it takes enormous imbalance, tipping points exponentially reached, to again experience the gift of a quiet center.

It is hard to imagine any gift wrapped up in death, divorce, disease, or any other of life's desperate situations. Most of us would ask what possible good could come from such heartache, and with good reason. Amid the hubris of such events, in the wake of such life destruction, hidden beneath the soiled and torn wrapping paper of a world turned upside down, one has to look hard to see any gift glittering beneath.

From an able-bodied perspective, getting a diagnosis of a terminal illness or winding up with a permanent disability due to a fall or accident would seem to have little in the way of an upside. Job loss, relational breakdown, or financial hardship are not what we would willingly invite into our lives. Yet as Cathy and I have both experienced, through such events on the parallel tracks of our own lives, we have discovered gifts unlooked for in places we would never have thought to find them.

For me, the revelation of gifts was almost immediate after my diagnosis. My physical senses sharpened for a time into a form of near synesthesia, where sunrises were tasted and colors were felt. I wrote in my journal, "The clarity of love is so intense, I almost have to check it like it is an energy surge. And I'm not talking about the symptom of extreme emotion (a symptom of many with ALS). While I admit that my emotions run stronger now, it is the blurring of the lines between my senses that offers such incredible clarity. I KNOW what is important now. I know that every experience has multiple layers, each to be felt and analyzed and kept. The autopilot of living from event to event is completely gone. Pay attention!"

For Cathy, such revelation unfolded more slowly in the illness of her father. But she too discovered wondrous gifts in the tragedy of her father's dementia. Her grief became a spur to deepen the relationship she had with her father. As Cathy wrote:

> In the midst of a loved one's decline, there is indeed a sense of urgency to do and say all that needs to be said and done. At the prodding of a friend, I wrote a letter to my father on the occasion of his seventy-fourth birthday. He was still trying to work through the consequences of his diagnosis. Disease and the specter of death can burn away embarrassment and uncertainty in pretty short order, at least it did for me, and I didn't want to wait to let my dad know how I felt. I wanted him to remember, while he still could, why he was such a special person and how he influenced my life. I wanted to thank him, and I wanted to put it on paper so he could read my words again and again, even if the words became difficult to understand someday. I never knew what he thought of that letter. He never said anything about it. My mother reported that he came out of his room after reading it with tears in his eyes. It wasn't until a few months after his death, when standing in a rented storage room, going through a box of his books that I found the letter. It was carefully tucked into one of his books. It was like a cosmic love note from Dad, and of course I stood there, letter in hand, sobbing. I knew I had given my father an unexpected gift. There are also gifts in recognizing and seizing the joyful or poignant moments and collecting them one by one, like precious stones. The smile of recognition, laughing at a funny memory, a hand held tightly in understanding as you say good-bye for the last time. These are all gifts.

As each of us has dealt with our own pain, ALS and dementia, this phenomenon of opposites has presented itself over and over again, revealing gifts we would never have known otherwise. We have learned that if we can move beyond the pain, suffering, and anxiety into a calmer space, gifts of clarity, urgency, honesty, understanding, kindness, self-reflection, vulnerability, joy, and, yes, grief might be possible. All exist simultaneously, past and future, yet mostly in the moment at hand.

Listen: a pronouncement like "you have ALS" or "you have a stage-four cancerous tumor" or "you have Alzheimer's" rings in your ears, obfuscating all sound. Yet, it also focuses you with the precision of a laser cut, forcing your attention like a slap in the face or a plunge into ice-cold water. There is incredible noise that goes with a terminal diagnosis, but there is also quiet clarity— clarity of thought, purpose, and feeling.

Would I have paid so much attention to physical disease in the world had I not been the recipient of the gifts of ALS? If I am honest, I have to admit that the arrogance of my own able-bodied existence allowed me to believe that I was in complete control of my fate. If I am honest, I have to admit that I imagined disability like I imagined being an astronaut—it was a theoretical construct, an unreality completely out of reach, and if disability came, it would be a swift end to an active lifestyle.

As far from physical perception as they may be, gifts provide balance in the topsy-turvy world of dis ease.

Over time, the gifts hidden in the challenges of managing dis ease are also apparent. In the final days of her father's life, Cathy noted:

> The small kind gestures and messages from others who've walked in your shoes and understand what it is like to care for a loved one as they decline and ultimately die are also gifts. Surprising and delightful and touching, they came from people on the periphery of my life, the people I never expected would offer help or comfort or solace, but who did and will always have my gratitude for it.

There is a perverse beauty to these gifts. The heightened awareness of physical vulnerability is almost sensuous in its presence. And the fatigue can be like a convex mirror, bending and shaping the images it presents into new realizations. For me, it reminded me of descriptions of vision quests. I wrote in my journal,

"The damnedest things suddenly become very clear—past pain, human frailty, regrets, joys, and visions, such visions of color and sound and wholeness beyond physical limitation. It is altered consciousness at its most primal. No drugs needed, alcohol not within a sniff, only the purity of fatigue washing over my senses." For us, to love, live, breathe, sense, and experience the tiny moments of this life take on meaning we can only relate but not adequately explain.

We have experienced the diagnosis, the disruption of whether to stay or go in both relationship and employment. We have experienced the loss of a loved one. Such experiences require years to rediscover that center, that space where all is well, that head of a pin where the angels dance. The consequences of great disruption are easy to understand. Not so easily recognized are the gifts where the small, trivial, carefully constructed sequences that keep us in an upright space are suddenly thrown far off-kilter, not by massive life experience, but by something so exceedingly small that deductive distance begins to look like the only way in which to understand their meaning. In other words, it's the little things that really get you, but it is also the little things that gift you. And here is the balance between disruption and its gifts.

Questions of balance are not to be taken lightly. For example, the balance between foolhardy and overly cautious could be driving five miles per hour over the speed limit. It could be the critical mass one reaches in deciding whether to stay or go in a relationship, or to move away from or remain steadfast in a place of employment. Most of us can point to certain experiences where our life's stasis was disrupted, where balance became impossible, where it was as if the universe had aligned itself against us. Being homeless, losing your loved one suddenly, being diagnosed with a disease that has only one, terminal ending—these are massively unbalancing to the overarching meaning of day-to-day existence. I used to drive five miles per hour over the speed limit.

I don't mean to minimize these disruptions, only to note that if balance will follow, balance is a gift in and of itself. Cathy observes:

> Dis ease also offers the rewards of honesty and truth if we're
> willing to accept them. They can look like the misfit Christ-
> mas presents you'd like to return, but in reality they are the
> best kind of gift. Honesty and truth are the birth parents of
> freedom. The honesty that spurs one to walk away from the
> wreckage of a marriage or the truth carefully concealed for
> years because of some shameful experience, finally revealed,
> can heal a wounded soul.

Honesty begets urgency. I have likened ALS to death by a thousand paper cuts. I try not to dwell on this aspect, the progressive
weakening of my body, but I know it is there. This causes a sense
of urgency for this life with these capabilities, in preparation for
the next life that is less physically able. It isn't enough to work.
It isn't enough to love my family. It isn't enough to connect with
friends. It needs to be done with passion, abandon, love, and
light. There is no time to hold grudges, be afraid, and not forgive.
There is no time for games. There really are places to go, people
to see, and things to do, and time is wasting. There is a gift of joy
and passion, love with abandon, friends who aren't afraid to say,
"I love you." I just don't have time for bullshit anymore. That is
the gift of urgency, and I am thankful for it.

The gifts of dis ease are many. Balance, honesty, empathy,
small kindnesses that ease suffering, even synesthesia if only for
a little while—all are gifts. But the gifts exceed the sum of the
good things. They are also the hard parts, and they remind us
that even if there were a world without pain and suffering, there
is a need to live the gift that life truly is.

And you don't need a fire department to realize the urgency
of these gifts.

10

HAPPY ANNIVERSARY

The first installment of the Minnesota Public Radio series of conversations with Bruce was broadcast on the one-year anniversary of his diagnosis. In hindsight, that was probably too cruel a date to thrust him into the public spotlight when he and his family already had so many reminders of how life had changed in the twelve months since hearing that awful news. Now, a radio and Internet audience was privy to his pain.

Some people might have fallen into a funk on such a somber anniversary, and to do so would be understandable. But later that evening, Bruce and his wife, Ev, went out to dinner, even ordering champagne to toast a year of life together in spite of ALS. They had made the best of living in a whirlwind year that included diagnosis, overseas travel, moving from their spacious old home to a small apartment, the purchase of a new condo, the marriage of their youngest son, the death of a beloved friend—and all marked against Bruce's inevitable physical decline.

For most of us, anniversaries are a time for celebration and reflection on things that make our lives feel good. The same can be said for Bruce, but in the process of acknowledging and celebrating his diagnosis, they also offered fresh interpretations of his life.

And finally, this most auspicious of anniversaries served as the motivation to act upon a moment he most regretted, and to be empowered through the act even as he physically weakened.

Anniversaries have always been important to me. I've tried to be an observant spouse, a caring father, and also a thoughtful person in my observance of these yearly events. I don't believe that I ever let the anniversary of my marriage slip by except for once. That was because my father-in-law, Evelyn's dear father, died on the day of our twenty-fifth anniversary, and it just did not feel right to celebrate a quarter century of life together in the face of eighty-seven years come to an end. And of course, on their birthdays, our sons thought we were celebrating their accomplishment of another year. But I think secretly we were celebrating the fact that we had managed to bring such remarkable young men into the world without messing up too badly. Any parent would understand that sentiment.

Ev's dad knew the concept of anniversary in a way that was much deeper than just marking another year. On board the USS *San Francisco* on December 7, 1941, he witnessed the crippling of an entire fleet and knew in his heart that he survived for some greater purpose. His contemporaries have been called the great-est generation, and while I am not sure if that is true, I know that he was a great man. I am sure that each December 7, he paused for just a moment to remember lost comrades and the gift of his life in the face of his very possible death. On the year of the sixtieth anniversary of the attack on Pearl Harbor, our entire family went to Hawaii with him to witness the significance of six decades past. Of greater meaning to me on that day was the way that he stood quietly and erect, head slightly bowed, in front of the memorial listing the names of those who died. Like so many veterans of his time, he talked about the good times in the navy and never much about the bad, yet on this day we could feel his grief and wonder at the turns his life had made.

In my previous life, anniversaries always served the purpose of providing some kind of road marker on the trip I was taking. I used the "life as a journey" metaphor way too loosely at the time.

I knew that my path was wide open, and I was in charge of my choices and ultimately my destiny—at least that's what I thought.

Now in this life, I have banished the metaphoric "journey" from any description of my existence. It is too easy, with too many lazy markers such as road signs and highways and paths and wrong turns, so that it has become a parody of itself, and it really does not capture the complexity of living with dis ease, ALS, a real life complicated by so many losses and equal gains. So to write about anniversaries is like dipping one's toe into the crocodile-infested waters of the "life is a journey" river, hoping that you won't be eaten alive. And while I believe the metaphor does not rise up to just how complicated life can be, the power of anniversaries in birth and rebirth as we live our lives cannot be denied.

This isn't a journey. This is life, and anniversaries become important when the changes are profound.

The most significant anniversaries are those in which we are born again. The concept of a second birth is unfortunately mostly associated with conservative Christianity, but it can be used to describe any number of mind-boggling, body-rocking, spiritual events—falling in love, intellectual discovery, overcoming doubt or despair—all of these and so much more could be described as being born again. My diagnosis of ALS was a second birth worthy of celebration and despair, but it wasn't my only ALS anniversary. To me, the most significant anniversaries compel us by their choices. Somewhere in the three months that followed my diagnosis, I realized that I had swallowed the lie of the medical model. My disease would have no cure, and I would die well before the time I believed appropriate. The choice was not whether or not I would be cured, but would I be saved. This is the anniversary—when I realized that in embracing my illness, I would be saved, and in rejecting it, I would be lost—that I prefer to celebrate.

My sister-in-law, a true born-again Christian, gets this. We share the same status if not the same circumstances. I do not have to explain to her how coming face-to-face with the choices of dis ease made me the person that I am. She gets it, because she faced down her own choices and arrived in much the same place, except Jesus serves as her dis ease choice. I would guess that such an observation would call you out, catch you by surprise. But just think about it, and you can see that for both of us there is a central choice and that choice defines our lives. It is why I love her so much. She gets me, and in many ways she doesn't even know it. But I do. I really do.

So how does one mark the anniversary of something like the day of disease diagnosis? You can imagine the swirl. It is truly an out-of-body experience. One year later, I hovered over the moment of truth, visually aware of the tendrils of clues curling their way from my memories to that neurologist's office. I could see the walk when Ev said my gait sounded funny, the day I stopped riding a bike to work, the evening I fell at a Minneapolis theater, the fall on the streets of New Orleans, and of course, the diagnosis appointment itself. For the past three and a half years, each of these events played over and over in my mind, confusing themselves with my present condition and future fears. I probably shouldn't have turned my attention this way, but I always celebrated anniversaries, so why should this one be different?

One of the nagging questions I asked myself is about the role that naming took in my progression. I asked Ev if she thought I suddenly "got worse" once I had a name for my diagnosis. She reminded me that she really took it on the chin when we got the news, almost immediately getting sick and staying that way for the better part of a month. I didn't need to be reminded. She privately worried, spoke fears only to the walls, constructed secretive Google searches matching symptoms with disease names, just as I did. Now, there was a name, an identity straight out of the 1930s, and the emptiness spawned by a neurologist unable to comprehend compassion except as something that might get in the way of a carefully crafted medical identity. Why ask if naming made things worse? It seemed to exacerbate the condition at the time. I felt that with the name ALS, I was suddenly hyperfatigued, hyperweak, hypervulnerable.

I suppose that implicit in questioning the role of naming in disease's progression is whether the ability to deny actually helped me to hold the symptoms at bay. I wondered if the discipline of holding it together was let loose by the diagnostic pronouncement, breaking down the denial and opening the floodgates of hypersymptoms. It is a plausible hypothesis. We know the mind can do powerful things, so much so that we control for the placebo effect. The mind convinces the body to take some measure of betterment, because the betterment is supposed to happen. Sometimes I wonder if my belief that I was just dealing with stress or a pinched nerve held physical symptoms off. Did they suddenly appear upon my participation in the great naming convention of ALS diagnosis?

My greatest regret since my diagnosis was the diagnosis event itself. I allowed a situation to take place that was harmful to the people I love the most. It took me three years to figure out the post-traumatic stress of this event, but I did, and once I did, I knew I had to go back. This would be a different type of meeting, one in which I would hold all of the secret information leading to my sharing at the diagnosis with one who represented a sick medical establishment. It would require every ounce of leadership skill, educative energy, and dis ease learning that I could muster. It would require that I go back with no expectations of the neurologist who rendered my diagnosis, and total expectation of myself who received.

So I made an appointment and met with the neurologist.

I met with him to make the case in every way I knew for a more humane, a more sensitive, a more holy and human act than what I had experienced. I met with him to say what I regretted not saying: that how one reads the script might be more important than the script. I met with him to help him see that great privilege, granted in a life-changing moment, requires far more creativity and imagination than is available in a strict reading of a perceived protocol. I met with him, and the result was predictable—he was defensive, and I pressed the advantages of ALS. Yet in the end, I hope that because I met with him, he will hear my voice the next time and the next that the holy experience of diagnosis is presented. And I know that by meeting with him, I am better now.

The circle for me was closed, and the power of anniversaries now realized its potential.

I cannot help but celebrate the anniversaries of my life. I still see the day when my one true love and I joined our lives in a reckless tumble forward into the future. I still carry the most minute of details of the days my sons were born. I still play over and over the day we knew we would embark on the great overseas teaching adventure, and I can easily relive the day we returned home to teach in Minnesota. Each morning I am greeted by the presence of ALS in my life. I would not have chosen this way, but it was the choice I was given, and I celebrate the life I have received by choosing to embrace dis ease.

As I head into my death, the anniversary of my rebirth remains, washing over me, rocking me with its choices, and I marvel at what it takes to move from this life into the next.

II

FAITH, PART II
It's Your Choice

I'm still grieving the loss of my dad. Fritz Wurzer died on a bitterly cold morning in March 2014, just as the sun was coloring the sky pink and mauve and gold as it came up over Lake Superior.

Dad always was a morning person.

He was not, however, a person given to mourning. If my father had grieved the loss of his memory or his increasing inability to walk and talk, it was hard to discern. He was a stoic guy. I can count on one hand the times I ever saw him cry—grief for him was likely disguised as anger. He'd get mad, growling and cussing, as he tried to move rubbery legs, hanging onto a walker, willing each foot to move forward, exhausted by the effort. He used to walk for miles just for the exercise.

I mourn his death and always will. Grief sneaks up on me at the oddest of moments, hot tears leak out if only for a minute or two.

Those who have lost loved ones to Alzheimer's grieve the loss of the person they knew before distinctive personality and memory were snatched away. They are understandably angry and incredibly sad that their loved one slowly morphs into someone unrecognizable.

I think of my dad as a younger man and recall fond memories, but I also learned to accept who he was during the course of his disease. At his core, he was still Fritz Wurzer. Getting angry over his dementia wasn't going to help him or me. Denying it was a waste of precious time. Bargaining? Well, I'll admit to that.

Bruce writes about making "hope bargains" when he was first diagnosed. You do the same when you make little promises to the Universe, ranging from "Please don't let that state trooper pull me over" after hitting the brakes to "I'll start taking better care of myself" as you worry about a health scare.

Bruce's "hope bargain" sounded something like this: "I can handle this if it's taking just my legs. Please, I'll put up with anything if it is only my legs." My hope bargain for my father was similar: I had hoped his mental and physical regression would somehow magically stop, if only for a while. That didn't happen for Dad. It didn't for Bruce. The question is, with whom are we bargaining?

My father's death was mercifully fast. Three days of hospice care, though the process was set in motion weeks before. My family and I did not see the signs he was disengaging with this world. When told by the oncologist that he was indeed dying, my father looked relieved, almost happy. I think he understood. There was no denial. No anger. No depression or bargaining on his part. There appeared to be a sweet acceptance of his fate. It took the rest of his family a while to catch up to him.

I miss my father and grieve for his grandchildren who knew him only a short while. I am relieved he no longer suffers physically or mentally and has been set free—to where I do not know, but I have faith we'll meet again someday.

What is faith other than a leap into the unknown, with no real idea of what comes next? And faced with the unknown, we accomplish our faith through the too-human activities of constructing frameworks, points of reference, liturgies to make sense of the faith experience, litanies to be repeated over and over again that bring us comfort. Nowhere is this more obvious than in the experience of dying.

Denial, anger, bargaining, depression, acceptance: if you have done any reading in the area of death and dying, you have come across the five stages of grief proposed by the great psychiatrist Elisabeth Kübler-Ross. Her conclusions were based on observations of hundreds of people as they died. Her five stages make great sense to those who have faith that life is sequential and that the mind can be counted on for ultimate meaning.

If you are facing your own mortality sooner than you might have anticipated, the five stages become—in weird yet totally comprehensible ways—anchors from which you can explore this new aching truth. They give you something, a meaning to which you can return even as you move out from diagnosis and into the loss of physical capability, into the realization that what you loved to do in the past may not be possible in the future, and the overwhelming and gut-eating jealousy when you view others' seeming well-being. Denial, anger, bargaining, depression, acceptance may suddenly seem like reasonable points of departure and return, a faith statement, perhaps. But in reality they are just names, labels that overrely on rational analysis, lullabies soothing us into thinking that naming something is a way to control it.

On the morning that my dear friend in ALS, Paul, dies, my faith is strong—weirdly, not in belief in the afterlife but rather belief in the present. Soon Paul will move from present to past tense. He was larger than life, a storyteller, a yarn spinner, a man's man who was not afraid to say, "I love you." As I roll into his hospital room on a summer Sunday two days before he dies, I have faith in his presence and in his past. He introduces me to his kids by saying, "Bruce is a good listener, and I have a lot of stories. We get along really well."

Each of us would fulfill a faith in the other in our time together, in the truth that we could speak without hurting. Ours was a friendship built in the holy moments that only two dying men can share. We knew each other for eight months, but ALS cuts through the need for bullshit. We knew each other from the beginning of time, and we would speak with each other truths that only two dying men might speak together. We knew that we had no time for false stages of grief. Stages do not work with dis ease. Anger and bargaining and depression and denial are a luxurious comfort, not affordable to those who recognize the winding down that is life. We knew that in the end dying and living are actually two sides of the same coin, and if we were to allow ourselves the sloppy weakness of naming arbitrary stages, it would only harden our faith into the needs of the moment, sublimating the truth we gave each other into a litany of surety, a liturgy that accomplished nothing except to name the space we occupied together.

ALS demanded honesty, and that honesty was the greatest comfort we could offer to each other.

I miss Paul terribly, and his passing graces me with a faith that belies naming the particular grief stage in which we thought ourselves to be. Instead, we seized the privilege of being together during that holy time into death. He allowed me the grace given when the dying rally for a few brief moments, and suddenly conversation and observation and joy in each other become possible, if only for a little while.

Don't get me wrong: I understand how seductive naming can be. Dying can knock you off your center until the floor drops out from under you, the tablecloth is pulled like a magician's trick, and the question is, will you spill out onto the table, wobbling, stumbling, stunned by the reach of someone else's magical illusions? At such times, how could you not grasp for surety? The ease with which anyone would latch onto a psychological model of dying that creates levels and stages is perfectly understandable. To name the space in which you suddenly find yourself creates the hope, the illusion that you may actually have control.

But control is nothing more than a litany of applied denial.

Denial implies that a certain reality is too overwhelming to be accepted. It is no accident that Kübler-Ross places denial at the beginning of her stages. Denial begins the litany because the beginning is where reality presses down on our consciousness most greatly. Denial does not anticipate acceptance, and it wallows in the anger and bargaining that make denying so seductive in the face of dis ease.

A few months before he died, in one of our many talks after yoga class—low voices and murmurs and secrets and codes just between us so as not to have to explain our conversation to others—Paul and I spoke about dying.

Paul and I loved the fact that we could speak the truth of our condition without pretense, that we both had come to a level of acceptance that was complicated because we had so much life we wanted to give back. He said, "I'm not afraid. The heart attack I had ten years ago prepared me for this; I have seen the view from the other side." It occurred to me then that I had seen much the same view through the eyes of a dying friend, in visitations from loved ones gone before I was ready, in my own dis ease. Paul's experience was more tangible, allowing me to embrace what I already knew. We both accepted the other side with faith and each other's stories. The rationality of stages and frameworks breaks down in the face of honest comfort.

And it doesn't just happen with ALS, death, dying. As a teacher of leadership, a practicing leader, I have experienced, recognized, focused on parallels between the stages of death and dying and stages of change. It isn't hard to imagine a person whose job is on the line bargaining to do "anything" to keep the job. It isn't hard to imagine someone who had great success early in her career to be in denial several years later that the way she accomplishes her responsibilities garners less and less respect from her colleagues, her institution, and its clientele.

Many people I know in the latter stages of their careers and particularly in leadership positions blithely move along without consideration of the new births in their field. The dying of the old ways, when the changes they should have made suddenly come to consciousness, hurt them and anger them. And if there is acceptance, it seems more like a crushing weight than a liberation.

Both Paul and I could see the parallels between the stages of grieving one's imminent death with the experience of grieving imminent change. But our experience together had no space for such frameworks, such idealized stages of change, such empty religious habits. Instead, we realized that dis ease is not about stages or sequences or experiences exclusive of each other. Both of us had lost too many friends to ALS to believe in anything so simple.

When Paul and I talked, it was the ultimate act of faith in honesty and truthfulness and each other.

Paul was the incarnation of living into death, and as hard as ALS made life for him and his family, he was determined to be faithful to what we both knew. Our slow, rambling conversations—with no point except to take in and give back the love that two dying men could share—acknowledged the physical challenges, the mental fun, the spiritual acceptance we both sought to engage. We spoke of having faith enough to be open to our horizons, not closing off from the beauty we shared— grandkids, sons, daughters, wives, springtime in Minnesota.

Staying open to all of this takes enormous faith, but when you are open, you embrace the world as it is, life as it is, love where it comes, and death as the gift of relief it is meant to be. No reason for denial, bargaining, anger, or depression existed in our times together.

We both knew that we were going to die.

If you need some academic grounding for this reality, then turn to the great psychologist Erik Erikson in partnership with his wife, Joan. In their early career, they postulated eight psychosexual stages of development. Each stage was marked by a conflict—trust versus mistrust, for example—and the development of a virtue such as hope or wisdom once the conflict was met. What does this have to do with Paul, me, and Kübler-Ross?

I find great comfort in the fact that in their later lives, the Eriksons came to realize that wisdom was iterative and based on the ability to balance between accepting one's aging and mortality and viewing one's life realistically and without despair. The long, meandering conversations between Paul and me walked the fine line between accepting our own deaths and viewing the lives we had lived with realism and happiness. The Eriksons documented that at the end of life it wasn't so much the ability to name the place in life in which you found yourself, as it was to accept the life that had brought you to that place. Paul and I understood this, albeit more experientially than academically.

And now, I need to ask your forbearance for a bit of grim philosophizing.

I have learned to equate ALS with life, just accelerated to a speed difficult to process. In life, our bodies will inevitably age, lose capacity, become incapable of the things we used to do. No one argues that aging and its accompanying physical and mental breakdowns are the future for all living things. ALS is just the aging process exponentially sped up. The issue is not the breakdown but rather the speed and timing in which the breakdown occurs. From a faith perspective, ALS is proof that we are alive, that we have much to lose, and that to complete a full and meaningful life, we must accept our fate with a realism that is honest and truthful and without despair.

This is really challenging.

I began this chapter by suggesting that there was something wrong in overrelying on the naming of the stages of grief and death and dying. What I have learned instead is to acknowledge choice rather than blindly accepting the tyranny of observation. Our choice is starkly real. At a certain point in life, either we can be open to the growth and beauty that life can bring, or we can be closed and engage in the irrational act of parsing life stages, death stages. My teacher, ALS, presents the choice in no uncertain terms, not just once but over and over and over again. Each time the choice is presented, I am asked, will you embrace the loss and grow into and through it, or will you deny its existence in spite of all evidence otherwise, losing yourself in the process? Stages of grieving offer a false rationality that the process can be controlled. The faith comes in abandoning your self without precondition to the growth.

When Paul and I first met, I thought my role was to offer him comfort at a time when his family was not ready to face his reality. He would tell me that my words stated exactly what he was feeling, experiencing at the time. Now, after his death, I realize how egocentric that point of view was. I may have offered him comfort, but he could circle me back into our shared reality and show me what it looked like to embrace with great faith our shared future. Talk about comfort. You can see why I miss him so much.

In my pre-ALS days, I would have seen the logic in committing to faith and the choices that living presents. But I would not have seen the urgency. I would have thought that I had all the time in the world, a viewpoint that ALS happily pounds out of you with honesty and abandon. ALS insists I focus on the juxtaposition of loss and growth, how seeming opposites are really one in the same. ALS insists I understand that life moves into its own speed, forcing me into the choice of opening to its possibilities, even as I feel life closing down. With ALS, I have been given the choice of opening to its possibilities or closing into irrational denial, anger, bargaining, depression.

With ALS, I have been given deep friendship and honest faith, even into Paul's death, even into mine.

12

HANDBOOK FOR THE
RECENTLY DIS EASED

It may seem quaint and old-fashioned, but some of us still enjoy trying to find our destination using a road map—one made of paper and folded in that mysterious way that does not easily allow the user to refold it properly ever again.

Some of the maps of the early 1900s were not, strictly speaking, maps of roads, since there were so few routes and not many cars. In 1901, the Automobile Blue Book Publishing Company printed detailed guides for pioneering motorists. AAA did, too, and there were others. Because there wasn't a uniform road numbering system, and no route signs along roads, the early guides gave specific written instructions. If a motorist wanted to drive the rutted route from Mystic to Groton, Connecticut, around 1902, these are the kind of instructions he or she would have read:

> 67.8 mi. 0.6 3 corners just beyond small stone bridge at
> foot of steep grade; turn right.
> 68.9 mi. 1.1 Left-hand road between old house and barn;
> turn left downgrade; trolley comes in from the left.

The directions weren't bad, unless the old house and barn that had been landmarks had burned down, leaving confused motorists wondering which way to turn. Those early guides gave way to paper road maps, regularly updated and produced by oil companies and state highway departments, that showed the expanding spiderweb of roads that crisscrossed the country.

Today, paper maps are largely passé. Many motorists prefer to be guided by a computerized onboard GPS navigational system or perhaps a smartphone. These are the twenty-first-century versions of those original road guides, proving that nothing is completely new but certainly can take a much improved and updated form.

Maps offer a sense of how to get to a destination, travel guides a feel for what to expect after arrival, but, as the TV infomercial disclaimer truthfully points out, "actual results may vary." The same can be said of dis ease. Bruce's doctors gave him a kind of road map as to how the progression of his disease could unfold, and while the losses have advanced as usually seen in ALS, the progression has been unique to Bruce. His "handbook" briefly summarizes the wisdom he has gained along the way; it is not as technical as a GPS, but it is more valuable than an instruction to turn left between the old house and barn. It is a road map to be folded back by all who live with their own form of dis ease.

In the movie *Beetlejuice*, those who have recently died receive a copy of a book, the *Handbook for the Recently Deceased*. Since the movie is a comedy, the book serves its comedic purpose as an organized jumble of information about one's options upon making the transition into death. Difficult to navigate, almost impossible to understand, it is the source of much of the plotline for this bizarre and humorous movie. This *Handbook for the Recently Deceased* is my inspiration, but I am writing about real life, demanding both organization and compassion. This is no comedy, although I have found humor to be extremely useful.

I can only assume that you see change on your own horizon. Perhaps you are, as the handbook title intimates, suddenly aware of your own dis ease. Perhaps dis ease has suddenly rendered any sense of control an illusion. Perhaps you believed the right decisions—no smoking, exercise, diet, moderate alcohol, plenty of sleep—would let you live forever.

This handbook begins with the observation that dis ease is no comedy but a sense of humor is helpful. From my own experience, the unexpected to the unbelievable will happen. There is nothing to be done, except to laugh, when you are in a lift, dangling above a shower chair without a stitch of clothing, and your caregiver cannot figure out how to lower you onto the chair. So many issues of great importance and seriousness will come your way that any opportunity you can find to laugh out loud will be a relief.

The fact that you have not skipped the handbook is indicative. Invariably, life demands greater requirements than we might have thought possible, and that is the point: to suggest ways to make the impossible less demanding. I will try to be practical, but ultimately the greatest practicality is the attitude with which you approach the impossible.

And I hope you find a bit of humor in the process.

1. You don't have time for denial.

Be amazed at how quickly dis ease moves. Even if you have a so-called slow-moving illness, the progression is always too fast. Here is my experience. Within three months after I was diagnosed with ALS, it was painfully obvious that I could no longer negotiate more than a few stairs at a time. We lived in a hundred-year-old Victorian home, and it was eighteen stairs to get to the bedroom. I could not believe how quickly I needed to mitigate stairs. And of course, stairs were symbolic. There was no way that we could stay in this space where stairs were required to enter and exit, where stairs ascended to bedrooms and bathrooms, where stairs descended to storage and an apartment. And even though we had thought this would be our final home together, the symbols screamed a new reality.

On the day before diagnosis, our fantasy of the future included our big old Victorian house. The next day, I had ALS, and any thought of remaining in such an up-and-down architectural structure was nothing more than the wisp of a dream.

But at first, I denied the need. I thought to myself, maybe

it will not move quite so fast. I thought that my anger and frustration would offer enough sustenance to my spirit to deny the reality and force ALS to bend to my will. That lasted for about three weeks, until I fell messing around with the cats. When it became almost impossible to swing my leg over the bathtub to take a shower, I realized that denial was not serving me well.

The moment of truth is not a singular event. Rather it is a process of honestly facing the reality of your situation. Truth forces you to see, hear, feel, and know what you must do to make things as good as they possibly can be. Whether it is hearing your spouse tell you that he or she does not love you anymore or finding out that your beloved child cannot meet the hopes and dreams that you carried for her, whether it is your own diagnosis with a mortal disease or the bad news that travels swiftly upon the death of a loved one, you just don't have time for denial.

So get over it, and get on with it.

2. It's not just about you.

The shock of dis ease focuses you on yourself. You have suddenly come face-to-face with variations on the theme of "Life as you know it will never be the same!" And it is easy to begin to think that this is about you. But it is not. Your new status reaches far wider than you ever thought.

Think of all the people who know you, who love you, for whom you care, and who care about you. Each one of them will see this new change with slightly different eyes than yours, and it will affect them. For some, it will be permission to share their own dis ease, the cancers growing in their lives, the wobbly foundation they feel, in the belief that you will understand. For others, it will be an analysis of what your news means to them. They will calculate and consider whether they wish to grow closer to a presence that is frightening, causing them to see themselves in ways they are not yet ready to handle.

Still others will be hurt by the changes coming to you, for those changes will cause them to embrace grief. Perhaps it is a son or daughter, a wife or husband or lover, a person who has come to see you in a singular way—father or mother, brother or sister, lover or friend—all must come to grips with the fact that you will no longer be the same person they thought they knew. Each person in your life will have to decide what your dis ease means to them.

Perhaps the most difficult will be those who will inevitably care for you. When I was first diagnosed and I began to play out the losses I believed that ALS would bring, I could not help but ask myself if a lover could be a caregiver yet still remain a lover. To the credit of my dear beloved, we have found ways to continue to watch each other's backs, to be intimate even as our definition of intimacy evolved. And, to my credit, I have kept a close eye on how ALS has affected her, thinking to encourage respite and care for her own needs so that she would have the emotional and physical well of strength necessary as my ALS progressed.

I could have so easily wallowed in self-pity, ignoring the effects of dis ease on those that I love. Initially, I wondered if I would be able to offer any sustenance to my loved ones, questioning my own worthiness. But as hard as it is to believe, there is always something that you can do to care for those who care for you. The nature of love and care is that each shall be nourished by the other. When I made the decision to let go of my own horror, to recognize that ALS was not just confined to me, it allowed me to enjoy a love much richer than what I had even known before.

The opportunity is simple. Your dis ease will either open or close your eyes to the dis ease around you. If your eyes are open, compassion and love and joy are within your reach. If your eyes are closed, none of this will make any sense.

3. Plan the telling of others.

For many of us, the idea of managing information seems manipulative, almost like propaganda or advertising. But you will need to manage how you tell people your news, not to manipulate the meaning, but so that it can be fully comprehended. After all, if you are recently dis eased, your news will be very difficult for the people who love you and care about you. Managing how you tell people will help you ensure that those you tell can respond in the best way they possibly can. If you agree with the logic that your news is not just about you, then you will see how important it is to plan how you will share it. Who should know first? How should they be told? Might the telling harm your ability to support yourself or your family, especially while you are trying to understand the limits of your resources? Careful consideration of how this new knowledge will be dispersed within the various communities in which you live will result in positive consequences.

After I was diagnosed, I actually kept lists of people with whom I had spoken. While this may seem a little compulsive, it allowed me to marshal my energy in a way that I did not have to wonder who knew and who did not. This was helpful, so that when I finally communicated with the general communities in which I was a part, my church and my university, I had built a network of knowledgeable individuals who could help absorb much of the initial shock. This decision showed its value over and over again in the following months. My friends and family, with whom I had first shared my news, helped to explain both what it meant in general and my specific choices as to how I wished to approach it.

Thoughtful communication will most definitely determine just how human this experience will become. Thinking about and planning how you share your news with others must be a priority.

4. You cannot do this alone.

Even if you are introverted by nature, you intersect different networks of people—your ability to understand how your news changes your relationship with them will be crucial to the quality of your life. Do not underestimate the networks that are actually designed to offer support. What will be important is how well organized your support can be.

For example, say one of the local cancer support groups can help provide respite care, so that your primary caregivers are able to leave your side for an all-important psychological and physical break. How will you ensure that this does not conflict with friends who also wish to provide respite? The very nature of dis ease requires collaboration and support, belying the myth of independence.

One key that has helped us to coordinate our networks has been to ask a friend to run our scheduling of volunteers. We tried our own scheduling for about a year and found that we were constantly playing catch-up with information as people canceled and others volunteered. When our friend offered to take over, it allowed us to communicate very clearly with her and then allow her to make decisions on our behalf. Of course, one way to read this experience is as a loss of autonomy, but for us, it has been a gain in energy. We are grateful, and any loss of independence has been offset by the efficient and effective development of a very supportive volunteer network.

Your understanding of motivation and resource will be crucial. Some people will volunteer for the wrong reasons, playing out historical needs of their own that you will not be able to meet. Such needs are as individual as our own circumstances. You will come to understand that some who volunteer do so out of a sense of guilt for something in their past. You cannot assuage these feelings.

Yet, there will be other volunteers who are genuinely helpful. You cannot ruin your friendship with them because your body has stopped behaving, you are fatigued, you are unable to play the good host. Such friends will also puzzle you, for it is impossible to fully show your gratitude for their help.

In the end, we were not meant to do this alone. Our families will require support. We will require support. Know your networks, and some of the challenge will be made easier.

5. Get your house in order.

Breaking through denial and remembering that others are just as affected as you are not enough. Dis ease requires actual environmental shifts. The home that you have so carefully constructed is no longer adequate to the needs now emerging. No wonder denial can be so harmful. If the nature of your dis ease is such that it moves quickly, you will find yourself trapped by your environment, made destitute by the financial needs of the life you possessed as you turn to the financial needs of the life that is now yours. It is important to move and move quickly.

Within one month, we made the decision that we would have to sell our home. But by the time we had actually moved into a temporary apartment, it was nearly eleven months later. These things have their own rhythm, and they take time. Every day that you take to feed any delusion that change is not going to be on your horizon is another day in which you will find yourself in a place inadequate to your needs.

Events as simple as the return of a son or daughter are as complicated as a diagnosis is disruptive. How we live, how our lives feel is dependent upon how we structure the environment in which we reside. And that structure must be living and breathing, always accounting for our current life realities.

You can live as if your house is a museum. The museum that preserves the lives we had is a nice luxury. But for dis ease, a museum will only get in the way. You must structure your living environment to reflect the presence of dis ease in your life, and this means your environment must shift and change to accommodate the next set of needs and the next.

6. Assemble your resources.

Most of us live at the edge of our resources, and the introduction of dis ease is certain to stress this already uneasy relationship. You can count on this fact, have faith in it, know that it will be true. But it isn't enough to know that your resources will be stressed.

You must understand your resources, both monetary and otherwise. From a monetary point of view, what will be the effect of your dis ease on income? What expenses can you either lose or put on hold? What new expenses will be necessary because of your new status? And it's not just about money.

One of the hardest things to learn is how to receive. For me, this has been one of the most painful and difficult of all the lessons taught by ALS. I still find it difficult to believe that friends, neighbors, support organizations, and government agencies are ready to offer help, but the truth is that help is available. However, helpers require invitation. How will you be invitational? It will certainly mean a loss of some privacy, but the positive trade-off is that you will be able to give the attention that dis ease requires. The need for such attention cannot be overemphasized, if you wish to find any grace in the experience.

And if your dis ease is massive, going it alone is out of the question. People will be your greatest resource.

7. Expect the unknown—find your center.

None of the very tangible suggestions given in the preceding sections of the handbook is meant to lead you to conclude that there is a single given path for your dis ease. The experience is as unique as each of us is human.

It will be important for you to identify the experiences that ground you, center you in the moment, help you to remain focused on the task at hand. You will have days when the swirl of information and change and pain combined with the desire to slip into denial will be overwhelming. You may think you detect signals from the universe that will help you predict the onset of the unforeseen, the nebulous, the painful, the unknown. Perhaps you do, but a tangible concrete center will probably be more useful to you.

The fact is that none of us can predict with full certainty our life's trajectory. We know how it ends, but we are not sure of what it means. Finding those things that center you, yoga or prayer or meditation, music or reading or just sitting in darkness, will help you to remain in the moment when all around you feels chaotic.

And know in your heart that chaos is indicative of normalcy.

8. Know the difference between curing and healing.

One of the most difficult truths to accept is that dis ease cannot be cured. Curing implies that things will be brought back to the way they were. But if you think about it, even something as small as a filling in your tooth will change the way your mouth feels from this time forward. You have not been cured of a cavity, for the cavity still remains. It has only been filled, and in the filling is something different and new, something you'll have to become accustomed to.

Expecting a cure will only result in frustration and disappointment. But healing can take place. When I began to attend the ALS clinic at Mayo, my wise doctor said to me, "We cannot cure you, but we can treat you." I took this to mean that ALS and the physical loss and the psychological grief that accompanied it could be mitigated, made a little better. The stories from my doctors and my family could become stories of healing rather than stories of loss. We would find ways to tell them together knowing full well that there would be no cure.

And to be honest, that is the way it has worked.

Not everyone in the medical field gets this. Medicine is predicated upon a curing model, and that offers little comfort or solace when one is carrying a dis ease that is incurable.

9. Engage medical treatment with skepticism, belief, and the expectation you will be better.

This advice may seem contradictory, but it is not. You must remember that medicine and medical treatment are based mostly upon the scientific method. The scientific method seeks to test the idea that there is no difference between any given treatment and doing nothing. Once that hypothesis is rejected, Western medicine has some level of confidence in the treatments it prescribes. That being said, most doctors and other health care professionals enter the field for the most basic of human reasons— to offer comfort and to ease suffering.

There is an inherent conflict between health care motivation and the scientific underpinnings of health care. Science cannot account for the complexity of human beings, but it can search for cause and effect, variable by variable. Most doctors do not understand that science seeks the simplest answers in direct conflict with the complexity of what it means to be human—that science is skeptical and humans are hopeful. Thus, those of us with dis ease must negotiate the contradictions of skepticism and hope.

We must be well informed of the expectations and the bases for the treatments that will be prescribed. This is where skepticism serves us well. But once we have chosen to participate in a treatment, we must shift our actions from skepticism to an acceptance that things will be made better. Without that belief, we lose one of the most potent tools we can be granted.

The placebo effect is not a myth, and it demonstrates the power that belief can play in the healing process. As you engage with the medical profession, counseling, and therapies, approach them first with many questions, and then embrace with fervor once you have decided what will be best for you.

10. Have faith.

I have lived in too many different cultures not to recognize that humans must develop a deep sense of faith in order to find meaning in their lives. This does not necessarily mean faith in a supernatural being. It could be faith in human potential, science, the Buddha, a way of conducting one's life, such as the Tao or Confucianism. Even atheists have developed a framework of faith that offers them direction and comfort.

Humans need faith. Without it, we are pummeled and thrown from side to side without any anchor to which we can hold, and life becomes overwhelming. Like stones thrown into a container that rotates first to the right, then to the left, we are polished by the life that is given us. The rotation never stops, and the challenges will only become more and more difficult. It will help you greatly if you believe in something.

I do not mean that you should be irrational or a believer just for the sake of belief. Approach faith as you approach medicine. Be skeptical yet ready to embrace, questioning yet open, and for God's sake forgive your body, your relationships, yourself for the breakdown that you are now experiencing. Faith will allow you to build the attitude you will need. For me, faith has been the ace up the sleeve, the one thing that I can count on as ALS ravages my body and leaves me weaker and weaker, closer to death than to life. My faith grants me great strength and clarity.

As I think about my past four years of ALS, there are things I did correctly and things I would never try again. In this handbook, I have sought to boil down what I have learned to its essence. There is no deep meaning here. Instead I have tried to gather possible rules of thumb to keep in mind as you navigate whatever it is that has disrupted your life.

Applying the lessons from above has allowed me to focus on living fully even as my body is dying.

13

TIME TRAVELING

One of Bruce's favorite writers is Richard Powers. There is a line in his novel *The Time of Our Singing* that many of us who find ourselves buried under a growing heap of life's commitments and complications can probably relate to: "Time is just one damned thing after another." Beyond the exasperation and tinge of cynicism in that sentence, it is reflective of how many of us view time. We like to think time is linear: a sequence to be lived in, a minute-by-minute mode where the minutes add up to days, weeks, months, and years. The broader sequence is pretty simple: We are born. We live and we die.

We describe time in many ways. It heals. It flies. It can be saved, spent, or wasted. We whine about needing more time. That's the funny thing about time—it feels like it speeds up when there is so little of it left, and it comes as a shock when time appears suspended in transcendent grace and awful reality when watching a loved one's every labored breath in the minutes before he meets with death.

We use all kinds of metaphors to explain our relationship to time. "Time is like a river" is a personal favorite. I like to fly-fish, so occasionally I find myself thigh deep in rushing rivers, but even as I cast my fly by standing in one place, I'm always in new water. The river doesn't dwell in the past. Its beauty is in the moment, which is really the time any of us is allotted.

In his "rebirth" into ALS, Bruce has made it a practice to live his life not with an eye to the past or looking ahead at a certain future but centered in the here and now. This is not to say that his awareness cannot be drawn behind or ahead. In spite of his sense of the present, Bruce states that he is a time traveler.

When I first heard Bruce talk about time travel, I thought it was a sweet way to describe the gentle daydreams of an idle afternoon, but it is more than that. It is reliving an experience, again and again, as if for the first time. For Bruce, time becomes multi-layered and expansive, and traveling in time is an opportunity to examine and add meaning to the present through a deeper understanding of his past and his future.

Suspend your disbelief, and understand that Bruce has come unstuck in time.

It is Sunday afternoon, with a hedge that needs to be trimmed, lush grass overgrowing itself, and the annuals and perennials stretching up to absorb every drop of sun that they can get. Suddenly it is summer in Minnesota. A few weeks ago, when we were teased with the idea of warmth, the air remained raw and wet and cold. Today, it is as if the cold and wet could not possibly have existed. The shade is comfortable, and a breeze plays off my bare legs. I have foregone the orthotic to enjoy the unfettered dance of gentle wind and dappled sun, tree whispers, and birdsong, all playing out in this little garden against the civilized hum of lawn mowing and traffic and commerce and recreation. In my state, this is a day that you can only imagine at other times of the year. In my state, it is respite from the weight of realistic calculation.

This beautiful day argues for the truth of Kurt Vonnegut's famous line, "Listen, Billy Pilgrim has come unstuck in time."

Listen, sometimes I come unstuck in time, floating between the sublime and the energizing, the feared and the fatiguing. Today is time travel, back and forth between imagery, both frightening and delightful. Today, I recharge, leaving the future to its own paths. I can understand how easy it would be to disengage from all of this. Dis ease does that to you. I can understand how you would want this to never end. Dis ease does that as well.

My thoughts have been so jumbled of late. We need some good news. It won't come from the voyeurs in mainline TV news, even though they try with their feel-good stories and cute pet tricks. I appreciate the attempt, but it is feeble in the face of dis ease. This week, I am laser-focused on so many friends who hurt, so many with conditions that threaten life and lived joy. The lump in the throat, the carried weight in the gut, the physical pain, and the emotional devastation—all of these come to me as if their pain is my pain, their hope and fear are my hope and fear.

In time, I have watched loved ones wind down, and it is always their conscious engagement that goes first. The body has its own rhythms, and it takes it awhile to catch up to human intent. I remember my grandmother saying to me on the phone, "I don't want you to send me anything anymore. I am done now." It took her body three weeks to catch up to her conscious decision, and I still marvel at how she did it. In time, others will watch me wind down. I am unstuck—lumps and weights of hope and fear.

I wonder if I am more susceptible to time travel because the newborn summer is what I imagine when I need a space to recoup. Perhaps it is because these are the days I will lament most when they are gone. I cannot imagine living without them. Imagination is an irony that isn't lost, for even though these days inspire me, that one act of imagining is dangerous, fraught with emotion, wonder, and unknowable destinations. I cannot think of an activity as wild and in need of structure as imagining. I cannot think of anything that defies the discipline of mindful structure as the stream-of-consciousness musings that suddenly emerge into pictures of possibility, tidy yet unkempt, restful yet active. Time travel.

I float in this semiconscious state. It is pleasant twilight, back and forth between naps and reading, reflection and dreaming. It is relaxation of the discipline of living in the moment that holds fear and grief at bay, allowing conscious vigilance to dissipate. Perhaps I will think on the loves of my life, or perhaps it will be the professional responsibilities that I still care so deeply about. Maybe it will be the all-important decision of a crisp beer or a nice Torrontés with dinner, or maybe it will be to decide not to decide. I know one thing. Even in this semiconscious state, I have come to see the differences between what is really important and what a long-lost friend used to call "conversation while dancing." Dis ease does this to you. You begin to pull away from the things that don't feed your soul, or if you have to engage with them, you ask yourself why you are wasting this precious gift of life on such drivel.

In my own life, I find it harder and harder to take seriously the turf wars, the one-upmanship, the personal ambition over the common good, the street fights for (really, let's be honest here) nothing but toys. Often now, in the middle of these pitched battles, I am not really there. I hover above them out of time and out of body. As the engagement in meaningless combat over this microscopic patch of temporal existence ensues, I ask myself, What do we think we are doing? Do we honestly believe that in this striving of wills, we can acquire something that will hold off the logical conclusion, something that will result in ultimate victory? In spite of the fact that proof to the contrary exists in the priceless relics of the excavated pharaohs of old, we still believe that it is possible to actually take it with you. Timeless and yet timed out, they could no more take it with them than we can, but the hubris of human pride is hard to shake. It is easy to become fearful, to think that acquisition is what will protect us from the finitude of our eyeblink on this planet. It is easy to believe that the person who dies with the most toys will actually win.

Don't waste my time. I ought to be home collecting kisses from my one true love, celebrating this fraction of a microsecond in the history of this glorious creation.

My mother-in-law has Alzheimer's. My father remains undiagnosed. Both have been bludgeoned by fear. Medicine tells us that dementia is a medical condition, tragic and cruel and hopeless. But life tells us something different. Only the very old souls can time travel, leaving us mere mortals behind to ground them in the present with the touch of a hand, a physical presence that cannot follow in the timeless voids in which they move. Who owns the problem here? My father's physical body is in a nursing home, but his mind has time traveled to a place of great comfort, a boyhood home with fields and woods and ponds and an old farmhouse, where he is happy. My mother-in-law knows moments of great lucidity, where she remembers and knows what she forgets. Her comfort is in her conversations with my father-in-law, gone now for eight years, or in talks with her father, a person whom none of us knew. As long as we do not violate her peace with the club of dementia, she is happy in her time travel, and we are sad that we cannot go along.

Time travel breathes, and in its exhaled breath are the epiphanies of joy and love—the embrace of a friend, the smile of a loved one, the eye-to-eye exchange that says how much each of us is glad in this moment. So much, and it costs so little. In my heart, I know only too well that both my hopes and fears are in these breezes of time.

So I am breathing in hedges and grass, flowers and sound, the music of living. I promise not to go into John Lennon songs or even to be tempted by the Temptations. To time travel is no trivial thing. All those pasts are still in the concentric circles beneath our current place, and all those imagined futures circle out above us, shaped by the choices we make with the moments we are given. Listen . . .

I'm going to collect kisses now—past, present, and future. It is the joy of gentle breezes, of freedom from orthotics, canes, wheelchairs and from a body that knows more and more pain in less and less movement, and of being unstuck in time.

14

TRIPPING THE LIGHT
FANTASTIC

Bruce started doing inner time travel shortly after his diagnosis in 2010—but he'd logged hundreds of thousands of miles on nearly every kind of mode of transportation in the decades before. Bruce and Ev are enthusiastic world travelers. When they were in their mid to late twenties, they parlayed their wanderlust into teaching assignments in Norway, Egypt, and Thailand with plenty of exploration in a number of other countries before, during, and after those assignments. Travel for both was energizing.

In the spring and summer of 2011, several months after his diagnosis, Bruce was walking with a cane. Stairs were a challenge and required great concentration to navigate. When looking into a future that clearly included less and less mobility and a shrinking world, Bruce and Ev decided to take two more big trips overseas while they still could.

Travel for Bruce, Ev, and family was purposeful, but their journeys always left room for the unexpected. As Bruce has written, "Travel is a dish best served with plenty of acknowledgment of just how little control we actually exercise when we leave familiar confines, especially in a place never experienced before." And as he learned during his final trips overseas, travel and dis ease share striking similarities.

In the months following my diagnosis with ALS, travel loomed as one of those major losses I could see coming due to the progressive physical impairment, fatigue, and just plain loss of gumption that comes with disease. We loved to travel, with our modus operandi being that I would plan the itinerary and Evelyn would scope out the secrets, the music, the food, the dances, the looked for yet unforeseen, the delightful, and the just plain weird things that take place when you travel. It was symbiotic: the strength of our partnership and teamwork, the great gusto with which we approached the next trip and the next, always led to a sense of joy and success, even when things did not go as planned. The admission that we would not be traveling for much longer came hard, and I tried to believe that we could travel as we had before. But in the months after I was diagnosed, ALS made clear to me the uselessness of denial, and the endgame to our travel as we had known it became a necessity.

So we planned two major transpacific trips—one to South Korea to see our son Jon and his fiancée, Kirsten, and one to say good-bye to two of our favorite places in the world, Bangkok and Bali. Even though I was on a cane (and probably should have been on a walker), we managed to find roads not taken, elephants, and fantastic beings, and the blessings of dance and music. And along the way, we learned quite a bit about what was to come, how we would become, as we moved into the known and unknown that travel can bring.

In March 2011, we moved into our basement to limit the number of stairs I would need to climb while we tried to sell our house, and at the end of the month we headed to South Korea to see Jon and Kirsten. It would be a whirlwind trip for us. We would arrive on a weekend so we could see them immediately, would let them work during the week while we visited Jeju Island—a place that would be very quiet except for hikers, though in the summer months it was swarming with newlyweds—and then would return to Seoul to spend a final weekend with our beloved kids. Our first foray out of the country with ALS along for the ride was truly a road we had never taken.

Jet lag has always affected me harder than Ev, and the

fourteen-hour time difference between Korea and the States is particularly difficult. When jet-lagged, I often dream vividly, almost wildly, and my first night in Seoul was no different. I had what I have come to call an ALS dream, usually about some part of dis ease with which I struggle in my waking hours—for example, denying the weakness in my legs and wondering when I would no longer walk—and these dreams range from the surreal to the highly realistic. Our first night in Korea, I dreamed that the pressurized cabin of a transpacific flight had cured me! So sweet, so hopeful. No more ALS. All I had to do was get on a plane and leave the ALS behind me. I awoke, happy and thoroughly rested, with my ALS new normal gone. What an incredible feeling! And there was more in this "cure" than met the eye, for suddenly I could let go of the vertigo, the fears I held of the next step and the next and the next. The greasy congealed lump of ALS, wending its way through my intestinal tract, was gone.

And of course, all I had to do was swing my legs out of bed to realize that dreams are just dreams. I stood myself up only to find that my foot dragged, my arms and stomach and back twitched, and that was that. It was a cruel realization, but I still received a respite, if only for a moment, and it was energizing. And this is where I gained new knowledge—that the road less traveled and the old normal travel were not mutually exclusive, nor can they be. I now realized that it is in my gut where dis ease really abides. Partly spiritual, partly physical, always present, my dream cured me, albeit only for the time I was asleep, of the ALS and the spiritual, emotional illness accompanying my disease.

We enjoyed a wonderful time both with each other and our kids. But it did not come easily, and it required of us an improvisation we had never felt necessary before. We walked very little and were ever mindful of how fatigued I could become. Often, I spent time in the hotel sleeping while the others visited places for which I could find no energy. What a different road this was for us. My old normal always had great energy for seeing just one more site, one more and one more. Now, I found myself waving my family off to see what I could not bring myself to see. I was just too weak.

Almost everyone who has attended a high school graduation has probably heard Robert Frost's poem "The Road Not Taken." It begins, "Two roads diverged in a yellow wood, and sorry I could not travel both." Three stanzas later, Frost states that what has made the difference is that the traveler took the road less traveled, not the one that showed the wear of constant use. Frost's poem implies that we can go one way or another—either-or, the road more traveled or the road less—and I was mindful of that poem as we visited our son and his fiancée in Korea. But from our trip, I realized that traveling and dis ease have much in common that belies the forced choice the poem suggests.

I came to understand that perhaps the choice is a farce, for as Piper Chapman in *Orange Is the New Black* observes, how would you know one road was less traveled unless you took both and then later compared them?

Travel is as much a part of me as any body part. I've always loved it precisely because you end up living on the edge, in spite of how well prepared you think you are. Paradoxically, for Ev and me, our friends and family, colleagues, and others, ALS brings us to the fork in the road where before we would have chosen the road less traveled, but now we choose the roads we have traveled less. We have to care about the dis ease we carry, and we have to carry the dis ease for each other, so that we are not so thoroughly buried by our new grounding that we cannot get up off the ground. ALS insists on a less energetic interlocution with the world. When we traveled to Korea, we recognized a new way to travel—less breathless, more protected, more traditional. We became cognizant of the energy it requires to accomplish the next learning, knowing full well that we could not predict everything to come, even with great foresight and planning and a good itinerary.

Upon our return, we began to plan the Bangkok, Bali farewell tour. Once again, I set the itinerary, and we thought about the mysteries we believed we had yet to experience. The greatest mystery of all was just how well my energy would hold and my mobility would remain. We were still infants in the disease, and we had not learned to predict what was coming nearly as well as we would later learn. Even so, this trip was mystery at its greatest, for we would learn of dance and elephants, with the blessings of the oldest temple in Bali and an urban shrine in Bangkok thrown in for good measure.

Dance has a spiritual side, especially on a rainy Tuesday in Bangkok. Ev and I decided to access one of the mystical portals of the world at the Erawan Shrine, a place where people from all over Asia make pilgrimage to offer prayers for blessings, for forgiveness, for things that they think they want. And we were there, meeting a friend from another time, who had come to help us hire the shrine dancers to dance a blessing for the many that we knew who were negotiating their new normal of dis ease. And of course, this included us.

I should explain a little about this shrine. The actual statue is of four faces of Brahma, each facing a different direction—north, south, east, and west. It is located outside the Amarin shopping complex and the Grand Hyatt Erawan Hotel on one of the busiest corners in Bangkok, an area now known for its blatant materialism. The shrine itself was built to try to correct the bad karma that accompanied the building of the first Erawan Hotel in the late 1950s. For some reason, the developers ignored everything every Thai knows about how building a new building dislocates the local spirits of a particular place.

In Thailand, it is important to determine the most auspicious time for breaking ground and finishing up these new buildings, and Thais expect to furnish a new home—some type of shrine—to which gifts can be brought to keep the original spirits of the place happy. The Erawan Shrine was built because at the time workers were getting injured, and accidents were happening in a way that could not be chalked up to just careless coincidence. A shrine built under such circumstance will take on a power beyond any Grand Hyatt Hotel, capitalism, or dis ease. It attracts rich and poor, the powerful and the dispossessed, men, women, and children. There is an omnipresent cloud of incense, and the sounds of traffic do not obscure its blessings. Even if people cannot take the time to stop and pray, they still find a way to make merit. We have seen people drive by, drop their hands from a motorcycle or car steering wheel, place them together, and lift them to their foreheads to offer a hasty *wai* of respect to the holiness of this place. Of course, the fact that they do this while in vehicular motion only increases the mystery.

In this world, holiness exists beyond our simple perceptions, and in spite of all the noise and commerce around it, the Erawan Shrine is one of those places. In the three years that we lived in Thailand and in the numerous times that we had been back to visit, we had never done more than looked from afar at this holy space. But on this farewell tour, we brought offerings, crossing the threshold with incense and candles and yellow marigolds braided with jasmine. At the Erawan Shrine, you can hire Thai classical dancers for whatever blessing you desire. You then sit in front of the dancers, facing the shrine while they dance behind you. The music is live, the dancers are beautifully skilled, incense burns fragrant, and the numerous offerings given around the shrine make the experience uniquely powerful. The fact that you have hired dancers to dance a blessing on your own dis ease is not the point. It is that you are given the gift of sight and sound to realize that in the dance itself is your own dis ease's blessing, and that by calling forth that blessing, you can dance too, even when your legs won't move.

And we were blessed.

In Bali, on our final trip to this ancient and holy space, we stayed at an elephant sanctuary where thirty elephants from Sumatra were transported to save them from certain death due to the deforestation of their island. The sanctuary was a working elephant habitat, where the elephants provided labor and entertainment, and tourists provided needed dollars to support the elephants. The irony that Ev and I were on the island of Bali with thirty elephants outside our door was not lost upon us. Elephants are not native to Bali. And while I don't want to write about thirty elephants, I have to admit that our final visit to Bali, at least when I was alive, made us acknowledge a number of elephants in the room for both of us.

Thailand has an almost spiritual relationship with the idea of the elephant. Unfortunately, corruption and deforestation have led to a great depletion of the elephant herds, which used to be far more prevalent in Thailand. We would see from time to time a mahout trying to make a little money by bringing a small elephant into the city. Advertisers would draw on the elephant's hide, and the keeper would sell the feeding of the elephant to parents who had become so citified that they didn't know quite how to show their children the proper way to feed an elephant. And yes, there are elephant sanctuaries in Thailand, but for some reason the sanctuary where we stayed in Bali seemed more pure, less corrupted, less romanticized.

It was almost symbolic. Thai elephants were depleted and moved into sanctuaries where they had once roamed free. Balinese elephants (admittedly from Sumatra) had never existed and so were increasing the elephant population on the island. With a body that was clearly being depleted by ALS, I wanted to be in a place where increase was the narrative. So after three days near Ubud in the inner highlands of Bali, we made our pilgrimage, first to Mount Agung to make merit at the oldest temple on the island, and then on to the elephant sanctuary.

Travel and dis ease contain their own rhythms. Those rhythms are sometimes hard to discern, but upon reflection you can tell that they have danced across you in ways that cannot be ignored. I could not help but think of how just the year before, on the same island of Bali, I had fallen, probably due to ALS. At the elephant sanctuary, one year later, I fell again. And there it was, a life rhythm with a full year between two beats, marked by falls.

I cannot help but marvel at the symmetry.

All life moves to these rhythms, and our belief that we can control them is just another elephant in the room. I sought to deny them by forgetting that they happened, attributing them to other factors. But there is no denying the old-man, shuffle-totter of my walk on this, my last trip to Bali, a walk well beyond my fifty-five years at the time. In Bali, I fell first with the left, then with the right, a fall and a fall with an echoing chasm vibrating the deep harmonics of dis ease in between.

Travel inspires. Travel with dis ease builds frameworks

of introspection. Visiting and staying at an elephant sanctuary means there will always be an elephant in the room. My loss of limb capacity was not restricted to my arms and legs. The progression, one beat to the next, made me realize that if my body was affected, my spirit would not be far behind. The rhythm of ALS always ends with the same cadence, and that can be really hard if you think life is about winning, that treatment is about curing. Our travel only highlighted the fact that ALS and life in general were moving toward their logical end.

The only hope in managing the unmanageable is to heal the spirit, to leave yourself intact and full of life in spite of the fact that death will come quickly. The artistry required is a razor-blade balance between physical symptoms and the spiritual strength present at any particular moment of dis ease. The elephants in the room of dis ease that I finally came to face after a second fall in Bali were that curing illness is ultimately a lie. This is hard stuff to swallow both for caregivers and care receivers. Dis ease management is about barely managing, and at some point, you don't. That is a hard elephant to look in the eye, and yet it sat in the room and said matter-of-factly, "Son, this elephant says you are going to die."

Honestly, I don't presume to understand the way all things work. From my Western frame of reference, it would be easy to dismiss religious beliefs as superstition, especially those of another people at a shrine in the middle of a huge Asian city. It would be easy to dismiss my own reflections as the grief that accompanies a mortal illness. But the Erawan Shrine and the elephant sanctuary and the admission of weakness inspired a metaphysical response beyond dis ease. I know that I believe in the science of science, but I also recognize the presence of God, the power of beauty, the hidden planes of energy that move in and through us, and the peculiar hold that Ev has over me when she cocks her head just so and tells me she loves me. Go ahead and boil any of that down to the physiological soup of neural connections and hormonal chemicals, and I promise you, it won't mean anything except soup. I just know that each small step in life has multiple perspectives and that its meaning comes not from the face you see but the ground from which you perceive and the direction you face.

Frost identified the condition correctly: "Two roads diverged in a wood." But dis ease means that you don't get the privilege of traveling one or the other. "Two roads diverged in a wood and I, I took the one . . ." And my only answer can be: "that I found myself upon." The way of the elephant is the way of the shrine is the way. It is the way of dis ease, but more important, it is the way of life.

15

KILLING THE BUDDHA

During the planning of this book each chapter received a working title and a summary of what it might contain. It was this chapter that scared me. Bruce thought that it would probably be the most raw of anything he wrote. The title alone made me nervous.

I know very little about Buddhism. I did some prep on its basic tenets for the Nobel Peace Prize Conference keynote address that I moderated with His Holiness the Dalai Lama in Minneapolis in 2014. Buddhist teachings underscore that humans experience many different kinds of suffering; in fact, suffering is at the heart of our existence. There is little control over this basic fact. Control, the Buddhists say, lends itself to a good deal of human suffering.

In October 2013, Bruce admitted that he had a need to stay ahead of his symptoms and losses in a way that gave him the illusion of control. He wrote that "as I look back on my control rituals, it is clear that they lead to this point: the endgame is coming." As Bruce has discovered, control is a cruel illusion, and it vanishes as the end draws near, like the soap bubbles blown by a child.

There is anger, frustration, fear, and hopelessness even for someone like Bruce who has worked hard to accept the reality of his life with ALS.

We all carry around images of who we think we should be, even in the grip of dis ease, but when that image is of perfection,

Bruce suggests it is best to cast it aside. Only then will you find lasting peace.

If you meet the Buddha, kill him.
                                        –Zen Master Linji

A Monday afternoon, and I'm stuck. One would think that with everything I have learned from ALS, I might have learned to sail through stuckness. It isn't a happy place to be. On days like this I know how ignorant I am, lacking any special knowledge of the human condition, so that my greatest insight is how perfectly imperfect my humanity is. I know how close is despair, how mocking is my anger, and how frustration and depression circle like carrion birds targeting a water-deprived man alone in the desert, stumbling and close to the final fall. Slower and closer they wheel and turn, and I can hear them, the wind whistling through their feathers, dust thrown into my face and parched throat.

A Monday afternoon, and I am not yet ready to die.

When I was diagnosed with ALS, my first response—beyond my disbelief—was anger. I was angry with myself, my body, my entire being for the betrayal that the diagnosis represented. It was as if in just one day my wife had left me, I had been fired from my job, and my best friend with whom I had shared my deepest vulnerabilities had published all my secret insecurities on a highway billboard for all to read. How could ALS happen to me? I was furious, and in my fury I thought that perhaps I might find a way through this informed by anger, fighting until the last breath. It wasn't until a conversation with a healer from Hawaii that I began to realize the folly of such an approach. I would only be fighting myself, and bitterness would consume me.

It was my first meeting with the Buddha, and I responded appropriately, though I did not know it at the time.

This morning as I was transferring out of my wheelchair, I experienced my fourth breathing incident in the past two weeks. In these events, I am unable to catch my breath. I cannot breathe in. I cannot breathe out. And of course my body panics with each occurrence—pouring adrenaline into my system, flushing my skin with cold sweat, wrenching my consciousness into an other-worldly fear I have never known before. My poor caregivers! Can you imagine feeling responsible when an activity that has always been standard operating procedure suddenly explodes? I can tell you that there is no quiet place to handle the inability to breathe. When you cannot breathe, it colonizes your entire being. I was left so exhausted that I could barely hold my eyes open for the rest of the day.

ALS has taught me great wisdom. It has taught me priority, to love and forgive instead of to fear and forgo. It has taught me to value just how precious the human gift can be. It has given me great opportunities to show courage and joy and strength. But it has also taught me that just when I think I can control its machinations, I cannot. What I can expect is to be pushed beyond what I believe I can handle, even to the point of panic.

It has taught me to be reduced to a fraction of the human being I wish to be, afraid beyond all belief.

I am inexperienced with physical disability, like an infant, a babe in the woods, challenged by all that disability presents. But ironically in the world of ALS, I am now a senior citizen, a grizzled veteran who has now lost enough physical capability as to be classed as having Advanced ALS. Couple that with the fact that more than half of the people diagnosed at the same time as me are now dead, and you can begin to understand how ALS, in its inexorable progression, grants elder status so quickly. You would think that with this elderly status would come wisdom, but that Buddha has died for me.

Writing is dangerous. Writing peels away the facade I so carefully construct, like sunburn three days old, itching and scratching and rolling into lines of dead white skin cells, revealing the pink below, the irritation, the damage done. When I look at my writing from my first and second years of ALS, I see a sense of clear naïveté. In projecting forward, I knew that life would become more difficult. I knew that I would continue to face greater and greater physical challenges, and that the emotional baggage that accompanies my physical regression would strain my very being. Yet, there was a sense that I should make my peace with what was coming—because I must accept my fate, because I am handling it, because the alternative is so dire. But the truth is just how unimaginative I was one year and two years into ALS.

The fact is that I have handled nothing.

There is a lesson here. In the Chán tradition of Buddhism, a story is told of the master who is walking down the path when he spies his student. The student bows before him, with the respect for which the master should be accorded. And the master strikes him. The master continues to walk down the path. Another student is spied, only this time the student does not bow but continues to walk by, showing no deference to the master. And the master strikes him. It is a confusing story, particularly for us Westerners who have learned to value cause and effect, behavior and consequence.

But cause and effect require that we embrace a belief in control. And it is way too easy to believe such drivel. Our technology and our science are a vast improvement over the superstitious relationships that historically were the underpinnings of our earliest human narratives. But when we are speaking of how to structure a life well lived, believing that our destiny is only a matter of consequence will result in being struck, whether we bow or not.

The lesson for me is even more profound. Every time I think I have it figured out, the answer turns out to be one hundred and eighty degrees away.

Disease sheds capacity, and while that shedding seems far too easy, it is what frames each evolving iteration of loss that I now experience. Since my first physical symptom, I have come to realize that from time to time, I must completely reboot, shedding the old concept of what it means to have ALS like the old skin it has become, and embrace the new losses as progress— usually with some physical struggle and emotional upheaval thrown in. ALS has changed me. Disease has depleted me. I can mourn each loss, but I must not allow myself to become comfortable on the new plateau where it lands me, for that is not the way of life we are granted.

I cannot avoid the ultimate ministration of my master, ALS. Whether I bow, or ignore, or thump my chest in defiance, or cower on the ground in fear, I have no control over the blow except to know that I will be struck, and I must move through the pain as best I possibly can. I have not rejected the gifts of science. My neurologist has spoken of ways to control the fear and panic when the inability to breathe becomes the standard, not the anomaly. But a new reality is coming, and I will learn new faith in my doctor's healing, confident that we will find a balance between the control I never possessed and the consciousness I have sought to maintain, right up to the very end. And this new enlightenment will only work when it does, for my family and my friends and me.

In the fear inspired by ALS, I fear I have not acknowledged the dis ease that each one of us carries. I fear I have diminished the humanness I have been so privileged to witness. I fear I have forgotten to acknowledge the parallels of ALS and the human condition. I fear I have been less of a friend than I should have been. I fear my inadequacies as a father, a husband, a human. In the fear is anger. ALS moves quickly, far more quickly than old normal assumptions. I fear the speed. I fear the teaching. I fear the teacher. Fear is the Buddha I must kill.

I will meet the Buddha, and I will recognize the falseness of the meeting—and in the falseness will be my new truth, carrion birds notwithstanding.

16

THE GRAVITY OF IT ALL

At first glance, any form of dis ease, from physical breakdown to crumbling marriage to job loss, would seem to be no laughing matter, but those who have traversed those challenges say the difficult uphill climb is made a lot easier with a little laughter. Humorous moments occur in any serious situation, and to notice and appreciate them are vital, or the sadness and frustration will crush your soul.

My dad was a funny guy with a delightfully wacky sense of humor. His brand of funny was more Jerry Lewis than Louis CK. Thankfully, he held on to much of that playfulness throughout his illness, and flashes of his former self would pop up at the strangest of times and make everyone laugh, including him.

There was, for instance, the standoff in the bathroom, pitting my dad, who was sitting in a wheelchair next to the sink and holding a toothbrush in his hand, against a young speech therapist who was trying to get him to use it. She was earnestly, very slowly, and a bit loudly explaining to him how to use the implement and demonstrating the proper technique in an elaborate pantomime. My father seemed unimpressed and sat there holding the toothbrush. The young woman was getting frustrated and figured my father's brain was so damaged that he had obviously forgotten how to complete such a simple task.

She had a stack of flashcards with pictures of a figure eat-

ing, drinking, and so forth with one- or two-word commands underneath. She ran to get the cards, came back, and triumphantly
thrust one close to my father's face that read "Brush Teeth." My
dear dad read the message, coolly looked up at the woman, and
said, "I am literate, you know." To her credit she burst out laughing, agreeing with him, and the two shared a good chuckle by the
bathroom sink. In the end, Dad did brush his teeth.

Bruce also has a good sense of humor and especially enjoys
clever wordplay. Even in the midst of our often sad and serious
radio discussions, Bruce and I will laugh. It won't cure his ALS, but
it does help in healing both of us.

I have been thinking about gravity a lot lately. Perhaps I have
allowed my situation to make me a little too serious, and I
recognize that I have been behaving as if my situation was
overly grave. But I know an opportunity when I see it, and
I might be on to something here. As my body weakens and
it becomes harder and harder to lift my arms and legs, I have
suddenly realized that gravity is not my friend. Indeed, it very
well might be that my problem is gravity. Most of us are happy to
have gravity in our lives. It keeps us grounded. It keeps us from
floating off at inopportune times, especially when we would like
to remain in place. But I am wondering if perhaps my problem
isn't that my muscles are weakening but that gravity is exerting
undue influence on my movements, singling me out from the
rest of the general population and requiring me to find some
mitigating technology to counter its effects. All I need to do is
reconceptualize the issue from a medical problem to one that has
to do with the effects of gravity, and then maybe I have a chance
to solve this.

Thinking through a gravity problem means really delving
into the etymology of the word *gravity,* and I turn to the *Online
Etymology Dictionary* at http://www.etymonline.com. The Latin
root *gravis* actually means heavy. That seems to fit me pretty well.
Too much weight, heaviness of the limbs, caused by too much
gravity. My legs are too heavy to lift. My arms must be gaining

weight as well, as the pressure on them seems to be increasing. It is a question of *gravis*. As we used to say in the 1960s, this situation is really heavy. But heavy doesn't fully speak to my situation. It isn't that it is so heavy as it is that things keep migrating south. So maybe this is a migratory problem.

As you may know, there are now real ecological concerns for almost every creature that engages in migration. Birds are particularly vulnerable to the enticements of big-city lights. They mistake lit buildings for signals that it is OK to keep flying, or they fail to perceive that the windows of a building are windows and not the reflections of the trees, sky, or horizon—real images but dangerously not real from the avian point of view. They will fly until exhaustion or collision takes them down. I have to admit that the big-city lights have always attracted me, and I definitely understand the signal to keep on flying until exhaustion. Evidently a number of people in Minneapolis emulate the same, as the police come out at 2:00 a.m. when the bars close to get everyone talked down, to get them to stop flying. In my present gravity-induced, migratory state, exhaustion can leave me feeling that all I want to do is drop. But if I drop, I am back to the gravity issue, although I suppose we could interpret my southern migration as *gravis* to the max.

Another migratory creature, the gray whale, also experiences migratory difficulties. It seems that the subsonic, low-frequency signals associated with motors and communication systems are disruptive to whales' migratory paths, as they are often in the same range as the signals the whales use to guide them in their travels. This can result in the whales beaching themselves—drowning on dry land, if you will. This migratory issue really speaks to me, as I find that often I feel like a beached whale. When I get into bed, my legs are so useless that I really cannot move once I am positioned. As a mostly restless, toss-and-turn sleeper, I find this very wearisome, so I try to keep my sounds of frustration at the subsonic level. It is in my best interest as well as the interest of familial harmony that I not wake Ev. She needs her sleep, and this becomes much more difficult if she is awakened by the hypersonic moans of the beached whale migrating south next to her. In this migratory vein, I see that my health issues are more about a new state of being, and that identified, I am back to the gravity of the situation.

When we discuss the gravity of a situation, we acknowledge that it is grave, and in my case there is no denying just how grave the situation is. Since it is grave, it takes on other meanings such as "serious, grievous, oppressive" or, as the Sanskrit relative of the word, *guruh*, means, it is "heavy, weighty, venerable." But that puts me back into the consideration of the weightiness of my condition. To be seriously oppressed is to access all kinds of repressed memory. Perhaps this weight gain in my arms and legs, causing me to more acutely feel the weighty effects of gravity, is actually a grievous, repressive state. No kidding. To quote Dennis in *Monty Python and the Holy Grail*, "Now we see the violence inherent in the system. . . . Help, help! I'm being repressed!" At least I think I feel repressed, and when I feel repressed, I tend to focus on how grave everything is, and any discussion of graves conjures up all kinds of imagery that I hope is premature.

Unfortunately, you cannot have a weighty discussion about gravity without a discussion of graves. The Old English word *graef* relates to graves, ditches, and caves. Its relatives are related to the verb *grafan*, which means to dig. While this is a state of affairs that I really don't dig, I cannot help but feel that if I don't interrupt this overabundance of gravity soon, my situation will have me ditching this plane of existence into the trenched grave, *grafan* specifically for me.

But there is more to this grave situation, for it is digging into me. As gravity works its migratory magic, I find my image to be more graven than grave. My body is carved, dug, impressed by the weight of dis ease's gravity. And although I have never considered my image as graven, it is clear to me that gravity engraves me with its indelible etchings, testing my mettle or at the very least meddling with my sense of how much *gravis* is present. I find the entire situation totally aggravating, and in a justifiable and remarkably symbolic act of defiance, I refuse to give it the proper *gravitas* it demands. In total insubordination to this unjust judgment, akin to throwing tea into the harbor over taxation without representation (although I am no tea partier by any stretch of the imagination), I'm going to engage in civil disobedience and deliberately break the law of gravity. At least that is my plan.

Just as soon as I can ditch this cave full of beached whales and exhausted birds.

17

READY TO FALL

One of the important milestones in a baby's progression is when she takes her first wobbly steps. Gravity is a handy teacher, and falling many, many times is just part of learning how to walk, scraped knees included.

As we get older, falling becomes more worrisome. The Centers for Disease Control and Prevention (CDC) reports that every year one in three adults over the age of sixty-five takes a fall resulting in injuries that range from a sprained ankle or wrist to a broken hip or worse, such as a traumatic brain injury. Bad falls, the CDC bluntly points out, can lead to early death.

Falling is also one of the symptoms of no less than thirty different ailments, ALS included. Bruce knew something was wrong well before his ALS diagnosis when his legs crumpled and he fell, several times, leaving him bruised and a bit bewildered as to what had happened. Those falls led him to see a neurologist.

Anyone who has taken a fall, for any reason, doesn't soon forget it. In fact many people who fall, even if they aren't seriously hurt, develop a fear of falling. That fear feeds on itself and becomes a nasty cycle of limited activity, reduced mobility, and a lack of physical fitness—which in turn increases the risk for falling again.

Bruce admits that the falls he suffered made him more fearful and less confident in his body. So, what did he do to push past his fear? He took a leap of faith. Literally.

He now explains what he did as something the "old Bruce" would have done—fight back against the fear of falling. In the spring of 2014, Bruce took another fall, his most serious to date. That one had new meaning for Bruce. You could say it was a leap past faith into acceptance.

In August 2011, at a time in Minnesota where we begin to anticipate fall, I became fearful of falling. At the time, I had fallen a number of times due to leg weakness. Indeed, it was falling that convinced me, pre-ALS diagnosis, to see a neurologist. I remember how falling made me feel afraid back then, less confident in my body. Over time, I mitigated the effects of falling by moving to more and more supportive and purpose-built medical equipment, including the power wheelchair in which I now spend the majority of my days. And I also sought to psychologically change the meaning of falling. But the truth was that in my first two years of ALS I fell numerous times, and somewhere in the middle of my second year, I began to feel fear with each fall.

The physical effects of falling—scrapes, cuts, bruises, and depending on the circumstances, broken bones—are pretty straightforward. Luckily, my experience with falling has always been limited to the lesser physical effects. I have never broken anything, my pride notwithstanding, and anything that was physically affected required only a short amount of time before I felt whole again. For a few days or even weeks, the physical effects are there to remind you of just what can happen when you fall, the touch upon a forgotten place, the breath that stops at sharp pain, the scab present in the mirror and not even felt. The physical effects take place, and if they are not too serious, begin to fade. That is not the case with the psychological effects.

I have always found the psychological to be more profound. After any fall, a psychological chaos goes on both inside your head and your body. Breath feels shaky. Confidence has been disrupted, and presence is compromised. The mind is dulled by the experience, leaving one grasping for words and feeling at odds with one's assumptions about the physical world, how things work, your relationship to the broader environment at large. For me, the psychological bruising is a phenomenon from which it is far more difficult to recover than the physical.

I have never been a fearful person. Fear has always inspired me toward actions that felt incongruous with the person I wanted to be, with consequences that I later regretted. I could see that if I did not face my fear, as my physical body regressed, my spirit would be defined by loss in both capacity and capability. In ALS, there was enough to fear without adding a diminished spirit.

I think that autumn meant more to me in 2011 than it ever did before. As I awaited its truths, they seemed to symbolize my own truths, my own autumn. As I worked through my own dis ease, I found myself anticipating an autumn with a meaning of color beyond the simple get-up-and-go-to-work existence that accompanied the blessed ignorance of my temporary able-bodiedness. As I tried to be both realistic yet still empowered, the fall held significance that I struggled to comprehend, for I knew it meant more than just the changing of a season.

In August 2011, the unfortunate focus for me was falling. Falling is a bad thing, all too often associated with aging and chronic disease such as ALS, and resulting in injuries that can be hard to overcome. And in the summer leading up to August, I fell more than once, and it left me shaking, bruised, and—this is hard to admit—scared. Each time I fell, I admonished myself to be more careful. But in my heart I knew that it was impossible to put the full, 100 percent attention to walking or standing that disease demands. And this inability to always attend, while carrying the consequences of falling, became debilitating. I found myself holding back, cautiously seeking the safety of sitting, staying, remaining, lingering in the quasi-comfort of my own small space.

Falling makes you fearful. It can color all your perceptions so that keeping fear at bay, ensuring safety first, is so paramount that any engagement seems reckless and ill advised. People fall in relationships, tumbling down due to their own or others' weakness and inability to take a chance on honesty and authenticity.

People fall professionally, allowing their failures to define them in a way that makes it impossible to meaningfully connect with others. Fearful of commitment, afraid of being hurt, the fallen exhibit a dis ease of spirit shaped by their life's own out-of-control nosedives. And professionally, especially as a leader, to become fearful was to become timid, scrutinizing every proposed new idea not for its creativity or capacity or inspiration, not to see whether it might imaginatively broaden our sense of who we could be, but instead to accept the dullest of motivations, to see if it was functionally convenient. In life and in dis ease, falling really does have significant consequences.

In August 2011, anticipating fall in Minnesota, I also anticipated the autumn of my dis ease. I knew that this was no way to live, no way to be defined, and certainly no way to experience human contact and trust and vulnerability. Falling inspired meanings with a life of their own. In that summer, falling meant fear. Falling meant pulling back. Falling meant expecting others to reach out to me, rather than putting myself out to others. I needed to reconceptualize falling into something that while evoking fear, also inspired courage. I needed to make the anticipation of my own autumn a celebration of the moment when life lived and shared is beautiful, and shared beauty is a rush of oxygen to the spirit. I needed to take the diseased meaning of fall and reinvigorate it somehow.

So I decided to go skydiving.

Skydiving is no easy decision, even for someone with an absolutely healthy body. As I told people that I wanted to skydive, the reaction was split: half thought this was a "cool" idea, and the other half thought I was crazy. But I knew I had to do something that significantly shifted the meaning of falling away from weakness and bruises and mistrust to something where strength and healing and absolute trust were paramount. What better way to rework the concept of falling than to free-fall in tandem with a person in whom I had to place my life? What better way to rework my head than to make thirteen thousand feet the distance from me to the ground?

So on the last Saturday of August 2011, I met family and

friends out in the fields of Winsted, Minnesota, and I went sky-diving. The owner of the company told me that it was his special mission to get people who might not be able to even conceive of skydiving to take the plunge. He even purchased special equipment allowing him to help someone like me, quasi-paraplegic with no leg strength, to put my legs into the proper position for the dive. As we ascended to our dive height in a plane that seemed remarkably small, as he and the cameraman lifted me into a position that I would have struggled to get into myself, suddenly that rush of trust and strength and healing was in my face. And yes, I was scared. There is something inherently fear provoking about dangling your legs out the side of a plane at thirteen thousand feet. But I was also scared that I wouldn't do this very real thing of taking back my fear. So I did it. I put my trust in a very special person, who took the time to prepare me, to help me, and to finally get me to roll out of a plane and free-fall for almost a mile and a half. It was sheer joy—air rushing by at what seemed like the speed of life, gravity's arc pulling inexorably, yet defied by the simple complexity of a parachute deployed.

I was tired the next day, maybe a little achy, but I gained a new meaning for falling. Even though I was sure that there would be another fall or two in my future, I now knew they could not hurt me the way that they did before. I now knew what it feels like to fall away from the safety of a perfectly good plane, to roll over and over, only to be righted belly side down, air rushing past in a way that I could never adequately describe. And that memory, with the knowledge that a parachute opened and lifted me up into a meandering, slow, undulating set of turns until we landed softly on terra firma, cannot ever be taken away. It was empowering. It was exhilarating. And it was exactly what I needed to take back the meaning and to be strengthened by it.

After skydiving, after free-falling, I knew in spite of the fact that winter would come and that standing still held danger for me, I held a different framework for the world, for I fell freely. For sixty seconds, I was free of earthly bonds, free from fear, and free from ALS. For sixty seconds, I fell into the assurance that I can indeed do this in spite of my dis ease, that I can stay the course, and that fear of falling, fear of failing is unimportant. I knew that I could trust, squeezing every possible beauty out of this incredible adventure. I knew that I could overcome fear and that any impediment to my ultimate path will be shed like a human rolling over and over, out of a plane while his dis ease continues to fall away, freely, like the rush of air at the speed of life.

Would that I might have remained in this space as my disease progressed, but if there is anything I have learned in the past four years, it is that disease is not sequential. You can imagine my feelings when four years into ALS and nearly three years after skydiving, I suffered the worst fall I have ever experienced, and the lesson revisited itself. ALS continues to teach me that life's meaning is informed by life's experience, both psychological and physical.

I thought I had taken enough control of my environment to put falling into the category of been there, done that.

Power wheelchairs are very technical machines. From time to time, it is important to change the settings, update the structures, and adjust the mechanicals. This can take anywhere from an hour to four hours or longer. My favorite wheelchair guy is Scott, a man who understands what it means to be in a wheelchair himself, having used one for the past thirty-three years. He knows a lot of tricks, how to avoid sores, and ways to make the wheelchair more comfortable. What I really like about him is when he is stumped, he turns to his very knowledgeable colleagues, and they all put their heads together and come up with a solution. He is really quite remarkable, for he of all people knows that the space for people in wheelchairs between getting to where they want to go and disaster can easily be mere millimeters.

After my last visit to Mayo, we determined that I needed to get my chair adjusted, and I made an appointment with Scott with the understanding that it was going to be longer than usual. Wheelchair adjustment is highly individualized—what works for one person might result in pain for another. It is much more of an art than a science or technical skill, and the amount of trial and error required for this particular appointment kept me there for four hours. I was pretty blitzed by the end, but feeling confident that we had made the right changes, I felt ready to take on the world again from the purview of my chair. A little after five o'clock, Scott and I rolled to the front door of the darkened building, and he said good-bye. I rolled out the door, turned right, headed for the van, and without meaning to, got too close to a curb.

To use a hackneyed cliché, what happened next was like a slow-motion movie to which I already knew the ending.

I knew I was in trouble when the wheelchair started to rock. I tried to kill the power to it immediately, but I couldn't make the switch work. I saw myself rock right, then left, then farther right, and completely over, my 190-kilogram wheelchair landing on top of me, pinning my elbow behind me and pushing my head and face into the pavement. Luckily I was wearing a neck brace, or I might have broken my neck. Unluckily I was wearing a neck brace that pushed into my neck and chest so that each breath seemed slightly smaller.

It was a confluence of errors. Ev tried to stop me, an impossibility. Her phone was out of juice, and I wasn't carrying mine. The wheelchair place was closed with no lights on. And its location is an industrial park where very little traffic is likely to pass after five o'clock in the afternoon. I remember thinking, "So this is how it will end." My breathing continued to slow. Ev was pounding on the door and screaming at the top of her lungs for somebody to help. I was weakly calling, "Ev, just come and sit with me, babe." I'm glad she didn't listen to me. Miraculously, someone heard her, and after being down between ten and fifteen minutes, suddenly I had people all around me who had been working late.

I am so thankful.

Luckily, these folks know how to work with a power wheelchair. Between them, they were able to right me and get the chair back on its wheels. One of them used the attendant control and took me into the building to warm up. Another called 911. All were comforting and kind and very concerned. My first ambulance ride, and just to assure you that I was only bruised and scraped, the ambulance didn't even turn on its lights or siren. After an exam at the hospital, my kids and Ev brought me home.

And here I am.

I have no words of wisdom except to say that at this time in my progression, the shock is not susceptible to the breathless fall of skydiving. Yet, even at what seemed like to me the very end, my body still mattered. When I could feel consciousness slipping, I remained present in my body, physically aware in spite of the psychological shock. I could discuss with you the philosophical failings of Cartesian mind-body duality at this point, but I see little use for it. Flipping my wheelchair left me just a bit too tired and still very sore, bruised, and shaken up for such a discussion. Even Ev was bruised from the ordeal, a goose egg on the arm and a big hematoma on the leg.

We can talk about it another time, for my awareness of just how fleeting life can be, how narrow the tightrope on which those of us with disability roll and those without disability walk, how lucky and unlucky the contiguity of variables leading up to and following any event, is hypersensitized into a weirdly balanced consciousness. My lack of words is a failing of language, not of learning. I learned plenty in this particular fall. Needless to say, I am happy to have a little more time for discussion.

And Ev and I are not finished just yet.

18

THE METRICS OF
MEASUREMENT

Bruce is fond of saying that control is an illusion. We humans laughably think we're in the driver's seat, only to have some catastrophic event hit head-on, throwing us into a metaphorical ditch—a crumpled, diminished mess, dazed by the sudden absence of the control we thought we had.

Even when there is evidence to the contrary, I persist in thinking that I'm in command of my life, and at times, I'll admit (with all good intentions) that I try and control what's happening with other people in my life!

Bruce and I would often talk about my dad's dementia progression, and I would mention how I was hoping the large doses of DHA (fish oil) and CoQ10 (an antioxidant) would bolster my father's remaining healthy neurons and delay his growing diminishment. Bruce would patiently listen, offer some advice, and then, with a small smile, slyly ask how my grasping attempts at control were working for me. It was a gentle reminder from a man who knows control is an illusion.

When one is thrown into the path of dis ease, in any form, the thin veneer of control is stripped away with lightning speed. If it is a health issue, patients and their loved ones are sucked into the vortex that is the medical industry, and it can be a dizzying and

frightening experience. Despite the best efforts of medical professionals toward the goal of "patient-centered" care, many times the
patient feels as if he or she is nothing more than notations on a
medical chart, the real person lost in treatment protocols, clinging
precariously to the hope of an improved red or white blood cell
count, a clean biopsy, or a clear MRI.

The good news is wholeness and healing can still take place
in the absence of a cure—something Bruce discovered long ago.

It is over four years since my first noticeable ALS symptoms, and
I will soon be going to Mayo for what will probably be my last
visit to the ALS clinic. I say "probably" because I have reached
the point in my progression where very little is left that can be
done to mitigate my symptoms.

The logistics of getting to Rochester, Minnesota—combined
with how exhausting the clinic tests have become—make the experience well-nigh to impossible for me. For example, I need my
dear daughter-in-law Kirsten to accompany me so that she can
drive the wheelchair in and out of the rabbit warren of the Mayo
neurological floor—my hands are just too weak.

And the fact that the Tuesday clinic starts around 7:45 a.m.
means we have to leave the Twin Cities by 6 a.m. to be on time.
Because getting me up and prepared to go is anything but quick,
the wake-up call has to come at 4 a.m. to set everything in motion. When we first started at Mayo, we stayed the night in a local
hotel. You can see how blessed I am by family and friends who
try to make it easy for me.

Mayo visits since December 2010 have mostly focused on
measuring my regression. The ALS/Functional Rating Scale is
a forty-eight-point scale with twelve questions with ratings from
zero to four each. At the time of my diagnosis, my score was
forty-three. Now, in the summer of 2014, as I face what I think
will be my last months in this life, my score is fifteen.

A study from 2005 correlates ALS/FRS scores with mortality, seeking to make the score plus the time since diagnosis
predictive. From the study's point of view, the lower the score

the more likely you are to die. But from an experiential point of view, as my dear neurologist Dr. Jones has stated, many people are still alive when the prediction states they should be dead. I guess the scale is only a little useful when you get to my level. Or maybe my doctors don't want me to fulfill the study's prophecy where x and y converge, so they kindly and deliberately fudge its predictive qualities.

Each time I prepare for my quarterly visit to Mayo, I have to go through a conscious exercise of emotional management. As I consider my trip next week, I am mindful that on the one hand, I feel relief in the knowledge that I have come so far with such clarity and care in the treatments. On the other, I cannot help but feel what I feel every single time I have gone to Mayo; that is to say, a certain resentment against the measurements that mark what I had, the capacities I currently possess, and the clear regression of my body that will continue into the future. For example, since I started the active breathing support known as BiPAP three weeks ago, I have actually lost three full points on the ALS/FRS. A friend of mine once asked, "What happens if you reach zero on the scale, do you die?"

I am really not sure.

I do know this. Since the beginning, management of this disease has had a familiar routine. There will be lots of observations, pushing and pulling by neurologists and physiatrists, blood drawn, pulmonary tests, occupational and physical therapy info, speech and diet evaluations, and an incredible amount of information offered, although each successive visit leaves less and less symptomatology to be medicated.

In the beginning, my visit was a time of measurement and prognostication, and I needed to be sharp in spite of the fact that the ALS clinic is incredibly exhausting. The greatest challenge of this experience has always been to remain whole, in spite of the systems that medicine imposes, reducing me to a series of measurements and symptoms that are indicative of diseases' control and prognosis in an unending and inevitable religious celebration of the power of science.

I have become used to the clinical language of my doctors.

For example, if they ask me about a certain symptom, and I state that I do not have it, the line they use is, "patient denies having XYZ symptom." The language of medical records is one of conflict, in which doctors probe for weaknesses. As ironic as it seems, there is little space for collaboration, and when collaboration does occur, it is more about cooperating with the physician than about reaching consensus. And while I feel the ALS clinic at Mayo tries to shift the paradigm, the DNA of the medical industry is so powerful that it seems hard not to fall back into the natural way of doing business: imposing a powerful narrative over one's suffering, forcing patient cooperation, and reducing one to a series of measurements.

Don't feel sorry for me. But understand that measurement has consequences, especially when we reduce humans to merely the measure. I am thankful to have found healing in the love and caring of my partner, in my sons as they deal with their father's mortality as imperfectly and perfectly as they can, and of course in the myriad of friends and colleagues who have reached out in so many significant ways. But measuring up to dis ease still remains. It is seared in my psyche as I move into this quarterly liturgy of managing the symptoms.

Thus, even in the supportive environment of an ALS clinic, I find myself fighting through the reduction of self into a progression of symptoms, constantly telling myself that these folks have my best interest at heart. I have to admit to you that I am so tempted to lie to them, to tell them nothing about this symptom or that. I know this is a delusion to maintain my own sense of control, but it would allow me to say, "I am in charge of this person, damn it, and you can go play your measurement games with some other patsy!" I know I shouldn't feel so defensive about something that is actually beyond my control, but I have this old normal need to measure up to the old ways, to behave as if everything, every measure taken, was normal. And herein lies the insidiousness of dis ease.

We really do lack control. All of us. To make life simple, more predictable, easier to handle day to day, we have devised multiple sets of measurements by which we judge our own circumstances and the circumstances of others. And when those measurements fall outside the range of what we believe to be normal, a range of which we are often not aware, we create a new normal that makes us think that we can control these seeming freaks of nature.

As if we had control!

Bigotry works this way. The big institutions—government, religion—work this way. And this is the way that traditional medicine seeks to do its work. Our great institutions prey upon our secret judgments so that the remarkable, the extraordinary, the frightening, and, yes, the supernatural are reduced to their simplest forms, and we are the poorer for it. It is classic and so typical for us as humans to reduce our experiences into oversimplified descriptions that we have made the experience of reduction something of which we are not even aware. Traditional disease management takes this unconscious reduction and makes it a conscious act, making us believe that the simple explanation is the most true. This is why the process of naming is so powerful and so impotent.

There is a scene in the movie *Apollo 13* where the astronauts rip off all their health-monitoring equipment in defiance of the flight surgeons. Suddenly, they take back their whole humanness by refusing to participate in the vitals and symptoms reduction that the monitors foster. As irrational as their actions may seem, I understand the way they feel. Are they really in control? Nope. They are still in deep manure with a spacecraft that won't behave. But they feel like they are more in control because they don't have to measure up to the assumptions of the (so-called) mission controllers. The scene speaks enormously to me.

If you knew me pre-ALS, you knew an active, healthy guy with all the unconscious assumptions by which he was measured. Now, with disease, I am framed by the symptoms and the measurements held within ALS. To get the most out of my disease management, I must consciously tell myself not to lie to the team, that maybe some reduction isn't a bad thing. Because deep down, even though my spacecraft is also not behaving as planned, I need to believe that I too exercise some semblance of control. To take this on in a meaningful way, I have to feel like I'm steering the ship. It is the human dichotomy of knowing that ultimately the ship will go where it goes—because of or in spite of the exercise of my will—that in a way makes me feel I have actually influenced its trajectory.

ALS—dis ease—has changed me. I am both more open and more measured in my approach to life. I am more demanding of control, and I have less faith in control's delusions. I am much more conscious of others' perceptions as to whether I am measuring up, and I am much less worried about what others think those measures mean. Dis ease picks off all of those scabs, exposes all of those fallacies, and it reduces the superhuman medical establishment and the ordinary human day-to-day experience to the realm of merely mortal. Measuring up takes on a whole new meaning, and it is way beyond the meaning of the measure. In the end, the well-meaning clinic and the psyche-battering neurologist will both have to get it. In spite of everything, we humans are basically in the hands of something much bigger than ourselves. Any control we might exercise is control only in that our existence aligns with its ultimate purpose. I find comfort in this statement of faith, and as I get ready to start what is likely my last Mayo run, it allows me my own measured reduction—my symptoms into the wholeness of being in this world.

It really is the only way to measure up.

19

A DEATH-DEFINING FEAT

Journalists have one of the most interesting jobs on the planet. We have a front-row seat to the show that is life in all its magnificence and horror, and our task is to chronicle it all, to help it make sense for everyone else. It shouldn't be surprising that some journalists, in their final years, months, or days, have decided to report on their impending death from a terminal illness or their survival after a battle with disease. This kind of mortality journalism receives great public interest.

I remember listening to a riveting commentary on the national feed of *Morning Edition* from NPR News one February morning in 2006. I was sitting in my Minnesota Public Radio studio as I do every morning, waiting to do a local break, when I became absorbed by the voice of Leroy Sievers. Sievers was the former executive producer of ABC TV's *Nightline* program and a broadcaster to be reckoned with.

During his career, Sievers covered wars in a number of far-flung places, including Kosovo, El Salvador, and Somalia. He was with Ted Koppel and embedded with the Third Infantry during the 2003 invasion of Iraq. Sievers was no pushover. When he was diagnosed with colon cancer in 2001, he wrote commentary on the experience. He beat that back, only to have it spread to his brain and lungs four years later. After that first commentary, because of overwhelming listener reaction, he began periodic check-ins on

Morning Edition plus podcasts and daily blogging. His My Cancer blog was one of NPR's most popular at the time, and in one of his commentaries he deadpanned, "Getting cancer turned out to be a good career move for me."

Sadly, you knew you weren't going to hear Sievers again after listening to his June 2008 commentary, when he admitted the cancer had "exploded." He sounded hoarse and weary. Sievers died in August 2008; his last blog post was written a day before he died.

Another journalist, print reporter, and editorial writer, author Dudley Clendinen (formerly of the *New York Times*) was similarly determined to chronicle his demise from another cruel foe: ALS. Clendinen was diagnosed in November 2010. Shortly after his diagnosis, he met with close friend Tom Hall of public radio station WYPR in Baltimore. Hall works on a morning radio show for WYPR, and Clendinen wanted to share his experiences with a wider audience. Clendinen wrote:

> We obsess in this country about how to eat and dress and drink, about finding a job and a mate. About having sex and children. About how to live. But we don't talk about how to die. We act as if facing death weren't one of life's greatest, most absorbing thrills and challenges. Believe me, it is.

Clendinen and Hall began a regular series of recorded conversations called *Living with Lou: Dudley Clendinen on a Good, Short Life*. Dudley dubbed the disease "Lou" as a nod to 1930s baseball star Lou Gehrig, for whom the disease is named. Hall would almost always start each of their conversations with "So Dudley, how's Lou doing?"

The WYPR series ran from February 2011 to January 2012, until listeners could no longer understand Clendinen. The writer had a form of ALS that began in his facial muscles and quickly affected his speech. I stumbled on this series of conversations in 2013 and was surprised they had occurred. I knew of Clendinen and his writing because of a specific op-ed piece he had authored in the *New York Times* in July 2011 regarding his advancing disease. The post drew immediate public reaction and led to another article in the *New York Times* by David Brooks, which continued to fan the fallout. Both articles sparked a stinging response from Bruce at the time.

In the middle of July 2011, Ev and I boarded a Thai Air flight from Denpasar, Bali, to Bangkok. On the plane, I picked up a copy of the *International Herald Tribune* and devoured it for the news, as we had been largely out of touch for the past week. I finally turned to the opinion page, and there under the title "The Good Short Life" was a beautifully written piece by Dudley Clendinen, former reporter for the *New York Times*. Clendinen had ALS.

Diagnosed one month before me, Clendinen had a particularly aggressive form of ALS that began in his facial muscles and progressed to the point where his speech was now affected. He had decided to kill himself before the disease progressed beyond a point where he could not actually physically do the deed for himself. At least that is what he said in the article, having determined that the cost/benefit ratio of staying alive on a vent with the need for twenty-four-hour monitoring, using a PEG tube to be fed, and being unable to be anything but "a conscious but motionless, mute, withered, incontinent mummy of my former self" was not worth it. Clendinen certainly voiced the fears that all of us PALS (People with ALS) have. This is a cruel disease, and none of us relishes the disabled future it holds for us.

I unequivocally support and supported Clendinen's right to determine his own path, but even now I am most sensitive to what may be the unintended consequences of his writing. What Clendinen did is offer a remarkably sensible and extremely able-bodied argument about how we ought to do debilitating, chronic disease. His writing reached out to able-bodied readers in a way that was easily accepted—without real questioning—as remarkably logical. I cannot help but appreciate this soft-spoken, Southern gentleman for raising the questions of how we die, and if you get a chance to listen to his podcasts, you will find his manner and thinking quite compelling.

But I am concerned about how the message is processed. In the end, if you are able-bodied this makes great copy, because you can certainly understand why you would not want to live as a "withered, incontinent mummy." By the way, incontinence is one of the few symptoms that does not come with ALS, at least not with everyone.

If you don't believe that Clendinen struck a chord with influential temporarily able-bodied persons, I need only to cite David Brooks, who picked up on Clendinen's article a few days later. In a piece called "Death and Budgets," Brooks cited Clendinen's "splendid article":

> Clendinen's article is worth reading for the way he defines what life is. Life is not just breathing and existing as a self-enclosed skin bag. It's doing the activities with others you were put on earth to do.
>
> But it's also valuable as a backdrop to the current budget mess. This fiscal crisis is about many things, but one of them is our inability to face death—our willingness to spend our nation into bankruptcy to extend life for a few more sickly months.

Speaking with the arrogance and assuredness of a temporarily able-bodied person, Brooks continued to make incredible claims about the failure of medical research. Those of you with a family member who has survived breast cancer, a friend or lover who has been able to manage AIDS, and each of us who has avoided hepatitis with the development of both hepatitis A and hepatitis B vaccines would find Brooks's assertions remarkably puzzling and even myopic. Rather than questioning an economy and health care system that can easily generate a cure for erectile dysfunction but cannot comprehend massive neurological breakdown, Brooks placed the blame for our overpriced health care on giving Grandma two more weeks of ICU. But he wasn't without compassion, stating, "Obviously, we are never going to cut off Alzheimer's patients and leave them out on a hillside."

Every once in a while, I have to express a cynical hiccup, and this is one of them: "Well, thank you, Mr. Brooks."

As a person with ALS, I refuse to take responsibility for the oversized cost of health care because I wish to meaningfully manage my dis ease for as long as I can. Just because Clendinen wrote with bravado about his own choice, don't start looking to me to follow suit in some misguided attempt to save society the trouble of taking care of us. Piss off on that one. Managing Lou is expensive, but not managing Lou is immoral.

There is some good that could come out of Lou, ALS. Clendinen could use his disease to help further our understanding of the illness. When he wrote the article, he still qualified for a drug trial, something for which it is difficult to find enough participants. And while his daughter respected and valued his choice, what about her choices? What does the loss of a father mean to her?

Clendinen overcame so much in his life. He was a twelve-stepper, a man who admitted that being gay required years of therapy to learn to love himself as he should. He revealed that his thirty-year-old daughter's inability to understand his choice was his one regret, and he wistfully hoped she would comprehend his need for a good death. Lou was one more cognitive and emotional dissonance outside the life he pictured he would live. I don't begrudge him his choices, but I now read these stories from a place that understands how easy it is to give up, to stop, to just say the hell with it, and to be marginalized as one of those disabled people. And that place is an open sore. If you start interpreting the choice to keep on keeping on in spite of enormous disability with able-bodied sympathy, you probably won't get it. Sorry, it is that simple: you don't know what the choices are until you face them yourself.

Clendinen's bravery was apparent, but I would argue that bravery goes beyond the desire for a good death. It is trying to live a good life when your old version of life has been kicked in the teeth—when you look ahead to less and less physical function but know that you have more and more to give. When your one true love tries to answer questions for a research study but ultimately refuses because the questionnaire is called the Caregiver Burden Inventory, and "damn it, you are not a burden!" It is plotting and scheming on precisely how to leave this world a little better place in spite of dis ease. And that is my message to

Brooks and my clarification of Clendinen, even though he probably would not want it. You get dealt a hand. What are you going to do with it—in spite of the fact that you are going to die differently from what you had pictured for yourself?

Let me tell you what I think a good death is. Above all, it is predicated on a good life, one where we take the opportunities given us to make the way a little better for others. It is looking for those opportunities in every day we are given. It is understanding that a good life is easy when everything seems like it's going our way, but the proof of goodness comes under the most adverse conditions, when the deck is stacked against us and when the most mundane of behaviors might require a day's worth of energy. It is knowing that we have squeezed every bit out of life, mixed it up, and given it back in love and care for the humans with whom we share this little bit of the great beautiful life that we will never truly understand.

It is not offing yourself with the thanks of a grateful nation to solve the budget crisis.

Clendinen's article forced me to look at my own motivations. I admit that a lot of the reason that I started writing my dis ease was because I hoped I might find a way to connect my new normal to my readers' current normal—a normal that I blithely refer to as my old normal. I thought I might be able to peel away some of the mystery as I experienced it, and my able-bodied friends could wrap their heads around the fleeting gift of their own lives in a way that would help them appreciate its light and not fear the darkness that dis ease invariably inspires. I hoped I could offer a way to predict the inevitable. Ultimately, I thought that if I wrote with transparency and honesty, then my readers would find their own way into their old lives, their own deaths, that would leave them not so much satisfied as accepting the fact that we each must come to our own mortality our own way.

I hoped that my friends and family and colleagues and others could see the need for imagination and consciousness beyond what we currently know and embrace the gift: "dis ease is my next opportunity to make this world a better place."

In the end, I guess I hope that we could see that this thing called living requires more than just doing it. It requires enormous spiritual space, so that Dudley Clendinen might have his good death, Bruce Kramer might have his good life, and all of us would understand that the difference is only a fraction of a fraction of the great unknown. Ultimately, it isn't about Clendinen or me, and I can assure all of us that it isn't about the actuarial calculations of Brooks on a sunny day in his *New York Times* column. It is about whether we used this gift of life to hug our kids, kiss our true loves, and bring a little beauty into the voices of night and day. It is about choices, and the choices are far more beautiful than whether or not we should manage chronic disease in order to save money.

Each of us has to find our own way toward something greater than ourselves, and I wouldn't trust anyone who thinks he or she knows the one way to that place. None of us has special knowledge. I don't, Dudley Clendinen doesn't, and believe me, David Brooks really doesn't. And therein lies the meaning.

Postscript

More than three years have passed since I wrote a response to "The Good Short Life." In that time, I find I have both softened and hardened in my reaction to the two pieces I referenced. My admiration for Clendinen has grown. I hope that my opinions previously expressed are seen as a reflection of my concern with how arrogant able-bodiedness can be, rather than as a criticism of Clendinen's choice for his own death. How can I not admire the man? In his obituary in the *New York Times* on June 1, 2012, he was quoted as writing the following:

> This is not about one particular disease or even about
> Death. . . . It's about Life, when you know there's not much
> left. That is the weird blessing of Lou. There is no escape,
> and nothing much to do. It's liberating.

Clendinen ultimately decided to have a feeding tube installed when swallowing became too difficult and he had lost significant weight. He said he was determined to finish a book about his battle with ALS. He died in a Baltimore hospice on May 30, 2012, at the age of sixty-seven. I am grateful for the opportunity to have gotten to know Clendinen a little better through his writings and his radio broadcasts.

And my feelings about Brooks? He is a columnist, after all, with a biweekly deadline to meet. He needed material. In my opinion, he did not think this one through very well. Such is the privilege that comes from a temporarily able-bodied frame of reference.

20

THE NON—BUCKET LIST

The granite grave marker nestled in the grass of section 2, lot 475B at Lakewood Cemetery in Minneapolis isn't terribly fancy—and if the grass is overgrown, the inscription can be difficult to read. What surprises and then delights a visitor to the final resting place of Clyde Earl Hagen, who lies beneath, are the deceased's wry last words: "My only regrets are the temptations I have successfully resisted."

Hagen was seventy-three years old when he died in 1974. His amusing epitaph reflects a soul who probably had quite a run in this world, and if we were to make assumptions, he likely gave in to a fair number of life's allures along the way. At the very least he had a good sense of humor. In words written in a garden of stone, Hagen gently suggests to his graveside visitors not to waste time. Live your life before it is too late.

It is a theme that makes for compelling marketing campaigns. Today, we're encouraged to live life large and fast and with passion. Reebok suggests we "Live with Fire" while wearing its sports gear. Pepsi would rather you "Live for Now" while tossing back its soda pop products, and Caribou hopes we drink its coffee because "Life is short, stay awake for it." Not bad advice, really. Life is short. Tragically too short for some.

The eyeblink's worth of time we are alive is why the concept of a bucket list is so tempting. Many of us have scribbled a list of the places we want to go and the things we want to do before we die. Usually these secret lists are tucked away in journals, but there are now specific "bucket list" websites bursting with ideas to jump-start the daydreaming process. While ticking off places and experiences can be fun and exciting, Bruce wondered, in a May 2013 blog post, if the emphasis on doing as much as possible before one dies is a delusion, deflecting attention from what should be more important in life.

If you are human, you have probably engaged in some form of fantasy about what it would be like to be totally free of responsibility. Such conjecture might be represented in a so-called bucket list—things you have always wished to do but for some reason or another have not felt that you could. The diagnosis of a disease that you know will kill you only increases the urgency of such a list. Whole tomes of cinematic misadventure have been based on such a premise, and it isn't hard to see how such a situation might speed up the accomplishment of those things you have always wanted to do.

When I was first diagnosed, I was actually asked by well-meaning friends, "What is on your bucket list?" Likewise, as I saw the end of my professional career close at hand, I well-meaningly asked my colleagues for ideas of the bucket list that I might help them to accomplish. There was a lot from which to choose, but the complications of desires that were sometimes at odds with each other did not lend themselves easily to accomplishment.

Sometimes, the complexity of choice is overwhelming.

The book *Until I Say Good-bye* by Susan Spencer-Wendel, a journalist from South Palm Beach, Florida, is premised on the idea of a bucket list. In 2011, she was diagnosed with ALS. She was brave, living and writing with chutzpah and bravado, and with that most human of desires to remain independent, choosing her own path even as ALS paved the road ahead of her.

I get this attitude. It is incredibly difficult to make space for dependence in our lives, especially when we are used to the independence that we believe defines who we are. She saw medical treatment as hopeless, durable medical equipment as giving up, and acceptance as her best choice.

In an Amazon.com interview, Cokie Roberts said to Spencer-Wendel, "Many people with your diagnosis would either crawl into a cave or go from doctor to doctor trying to survive a little longer. You chose not to do that. Why?" Spencer-Wendel answered, "The problem with a cave is it has no windows. And the problem with knocking on umpteen doctor doors is that there is nothing behind the door. . . . I am not giving up. I am accepting. . . . Also a major factor is my husband. I so want him to have a chance at another life. Not saddled with the weight of an invalid wife."

In the book, Spencer-Wendel says she decided to devote herself to a year of "living joyfully," through extended travel to see among other things the northern lights, Budapest, her favorite beaches, and the island of Cyprus in search of her birth family (she was adopted as a baby). Sometimes, she traveled with her family, and sometimes she did not, but her main motivation was to make meaningful memories before she died.

This was her bucket list, and out of it came a book and a movie contract.

Please understand that I have no problem with a person with ALS exercising as much control over their own lives as possible, even if it means hastening their own demise. Until you face ALS and own it as your own personal disease, I don't see how you can judge such words and actions. Until you face ALS, agreement or disagreement is purely speculative.

Anytime a person writes the words "please understand," you can probably predict that they are conflicted. I am guilty as charged. The conflict that causes me anxiety is Spencer-Wendel's choice to engage the temporarily able-bodied fantasies that come with the bucket list. In many ways, I suspect that most people would not even see this. What has struck me about bucket lists is that they offer a kind of "hall pass" to life: because you have a mortal disease, no responsibilities, no cares, you deserve it.

I don't think this is Spencer-Wendel's intention. She intended to make memories that would cement her into the psyches of her children and her husband. She intended to do what all writers must do. She wrote, eighty-three thousand words, with her thumb, on an iPhone!

And it is clear to me that once you have published something, it is beyond your control how it will be perceived. When National Public Radio *Weekend Edition*'s Scott Simon interviewed Spencer-Wendel's husband, Simon declared, "This book is so funny!" But Simon made this declaration immediately after asking him how he was doing and receiving the following answer: "Well—difficult. Every day I wake up, I feel sad. That's my first emotion. And then I roll over, and I look at Susan. And I realize that she's not allowing herself to feel that way, so I can't— and I don't." All that I could hear in that answer was the weariness of a caregiver who was trying to support his beloved spouse as she lived into her own death. And as much humor as Susan Spencer-Wendel tried to put into the book, there is also an overarching sadness always present when she speaks of her children and her husband.

There is no bucket list that will cure such a side effect.

I am reminded of when Dudley Clendinen wrote about his decision to kill himself because he did not want to become a "conscious but motionless, mute, withered, incontinent mummy of my former self." Clendinen expressed the fear that all of us with ALS secretly or not so secretly carry—that somehow we will become "locked-in," trapped in our bodies with no way to communicate, no way to engage, and, most significantly, with no way out. His bucket list was to control his manner of death. Spencer-Wendel's bucket list is partially inspired by her fear of saddling an able-bodied spouse with an invalid. The fears that inspired both are perfectly understandable. I carry the same fears myself.

But I wish with all my heart that such fear did not reinforce the outlook that being disabled requires some heroic gesture— rather than engaging with disability as a normal way that the world works. I worry that those of us who write from an ALS perspective may play into the not-so-subtle ratification that a life framed by disability can be easily judged to be less than living. I worry that from an able-bodied perspective, our stories reinforce a Temporary Able-Bodied myth that is long on issuing a hall pass for terminal living—no responsibilities, no problem—and short on looking at the consequences of such easy assumptions. I worry that any singular focus on the person with disease conveniently disregards the family, friends, and colleagues also affected by their loved one's illness. I worry about reinforcing the idea that life with massive disability is life not worth living, unhappy and unfulfilling, meaningless and unengaged.

So what is the alternative to the bucket list?

I think we have to lose the fantasy. Instead, perhaps it would be better to construct a non–bucket list of blessings and complexity and empathy. In 2009, Eric Lowen of the folk rock duo Lowen and Navarro participated in a *New York Times* perspective called "The Voices of ALS." Listen to his words: "The hardest part for me is the pain I bring everybody. The fact that my children have to deal with it and my wife, I wish I could disappear quietly. But it doesn't work like that. That's the most horrible for me." He continues: "I thought at first I was going to live every day to the fullest and not let anything stand in the way, but then I got a hangnail, then I got a stomachache. . . . life is pretty much the same no matter what and the thing that has helped me the most is a quote from a friend of mine. She said, 'We're all on a journey. You just have a better map.' I think that's the way it is."

I so get this it makes me hurt.

What seems to get lost in able-bodied frameworks is the message that life goes on, that ALS can be a life sentence, not just a death sentence. And while we cannot all be poets, Lowen sang ALS in such a profound way until he could not perform anymore, engaging in new life even as ALS slowly eroded the old life that was his. In his song "Learning to Fall," he wrote about his better map. He noted the beauty of new blessing, of still having time, of knowing where you stand, and most appropriate to ALS, of learning how to fall.

In the year since I published a blog about Spencer-Wendel, Clendinen, and Lowen, it should be no surprise that my own thinking has evolved. In particular, I cannot help but hold Lowen just a little closer to my heart. His wife wrote me after the blog was published and pointed out that his choices aimed toward being able to see his two children, and her three, all of the same age, graduate from high school, all at the same time. And he nearly made it. He didn't live long enough to see them all graduate, but he did see them accepted into college (all five of them!). In my own heart, I think I know what this meant.

There is no way to misinterpret the meaning of a person's life devoted to those whom he or she loves, Susan Spencer-Wendel's, Dudley Clendinen's, Eric Lowen's, and mine.

Now, as I wind down into the final days of my own disease, I am far more sympathetic to the bucket list that Spencer-Wendel sought to accomplish before her death, the good death that Clendinen hoped would be his, and the familial engagement that Lowen strove to realize. I am inspired by all three.

And that is the real point. We can either die while we are dying or live our lives to the fullest. But neither massive disability nor incredible bucket lists will be the determinant of life value. It is the non—bucket list of learning how to fall into new blessings, and somehow in the falling, bringing those that you love along for the ride.

21

THE WIDENING GYRE

A car's windshield and its rearview mirror wouldn't immediately seem like useful metaphors for life, but some motivational speakers and authors like the analogy. It goes like this. Notice how a car has a large windshield and a smaller rearview mirror. Of course the driver spends more time looking out the windshield at the road ahead. The rearview mirror is used to see what's behind the car. Think now of your life. In the book *Become a Better You*, popular media minister Joel Osteen writes that "the implication is obvious . . . where you are going is much more important than where you've been."

That depends on one's perspective.

It may be easier to leave the past in the distance because it is much too painful and messy to ponder how it may inform the future. Others find great value in mining the past for a deeper understanding of their lives today. That doesn't mean the examination is easy. Looking back—especially when one is living with a difficult illness or disability—can bring on waves of grief for what was.

In April and August 2013, Bruce wrote blogs about the pain associated with looking back at old photos of his pre-ALS life as well as some of his early writing postdiagnosis. He had suffered numerous losses due to the disease. Bruce called some of these losses "paper cuts," but they signified a snowballing progression of disease. A weak left foot unable to depress the clutch in his favorite manual transmission car led to buying a vehicle with an automatic transmission. A paper cut. In due time, a driving assessment found Bruce's arms too weak to properly maneuver a steering wheel. Another paper cut. Each loss stung badly, drawing its own form of blood. He has described ALS as "death by a thousand paper cuts," and that is a pretty apt metaphor for the insidious way the disease works.

As Bruce looks back at his life with ALS, he likens it to a gyre—a large, looping endeavor where a current event may bisect that of the past and both take on a fresher, deeper interpretation. The gyre is mentioned in the famed poem "The Second Coming" by Bruce's favorite poet, William Butler Yeats.

> *Turning and turning in the widening gyre*
> *The falcon cannot hear the falconer;*
> *Things fall apart; the centre cannot hold;*

But the center is exactly where Bruce tries to place himself. Neither too far ahead, nor stuck in the past, but in the only time ever really available to any of us. This moment. Right now. That center is a good vantage point from which to look back.

Almost to the day that I turned fifty, I experienced a phenomenon that many of my older and wiser friends easily recognized. I would get up in the morning, look in the mirror, and wonder, Who is that old man staring back at me? Or I would be walking by a bank of windows, and I would catch a glimpse of myself and not recognize the person looking back. As I have continued to age, this experience has only continued to heighten. You might interpret my nonrecognition as narcissistic, and I guess I wouldn't blame you if you did. Yet I believe something instructive exists in whether we fully recognize our physical selves. I had this experience recently when I downloaded pictures from a small trip we made to Chicago. There was one picture in particular that when it came up on the computer, made me stop and wonder if that was really me.

We spent our first day at Millennium Park. Chicago has a

well-developed park system along the lake, but when Millennium Park was built, it was highly controversial due to its cost and location—a park on some of the most valuable land in downtown Chicago. Now, nearly ten years after its opening, it is a place of energy and fun and wonderful amenities enjoyed by thousands of people every day, even in the winter. We spent almost two hours listening to the Grant Park Orchestra rehearsing an upcoming performance of the Shostakovich Fifth Symphony, enjoying the bizarre sculptures, and of course, no visit is complete without hanging around the great fountain that projects pictures of faces between its two monoliths—children and adults splashing in its puddles and standing under its bubbling waters. The whole park is meant to be interactive.

That day—lovely and sunny and cool for July—invited us to linger in the park, enjoying its beauty, recording the occasion with lots of pictures. Toward the entrance of the park, we stopped for a picture: Evelyn bending down to be at my height, me in the wheelchair, crooked, Buddha-bellied, hands tired from steering. I describe this in such terms because for the first time in a long time, I was surprised at my lack of recognition that it was me in the picture. Something about the picture projected what I think of as ALS posture—a picture that my subconscious has always seen in others but not in myself. It broke through my denial, spilling waves of cognitive dissonance between the body I have, the person I am, and the way I see myself. Suddenly, I saw myself with others' eyes, and all of those old feelings about disability and deniability came rushing back as if I realized my disabled condition for the first time all over again.

I guess I really am a TAB (temporarily able-bodied person) at heart. I just can't help it.

It was the circling gyre all over again—a point on the path of dis ease that I thought I had put behind me—only to spiral around to a deeper (or perhaps more superficial) interpretation of that same event. I thought that I had reached some semblance of acceptance—where this physical body is what it is, and my own self-worth is not a by-product of physical capacity's superficial interpretation. You can imagine how surprised I was, not just by the picture but by my own over-the-top reaction of shock and denial.

Usually I have my head around these things, and I am able to live within my disability with a pretty healthy attitude, but seeing that picture put me right back into the denial I had experienced when my ALS first began. And associated with such denial is an unhealthy self-esteem tied up in physical projection. I questioned whether I deserved the love and attention of my family and my friends, because, after all, I was not whole, I was not well, I was ALS personified—scoliosis, gut protruding, wheelchair bound, muscles deteriorating. Not a pretty sight.

All of this from one picture? Eventually, I was able to find balance, harmony—a place where I could accept that it is just my body, and the space that I occupy is far greater than the capability and capacity my body projects.

In working on this book, the revision of various blog entries from nearly four years ago requires close consideration of my narrative in dis ease—trolling through earlier postings, journals, and even pictures. And this has not been easy. Sitting inside any former blog entry is grief for some hidden reference, some thing I was able to do then but cannot do now. Inside every picture is an image of my old normal, even when I thought it was the new normal. Inside this book is grief for the teaching I can no longer do. Dis ease has taught me that looking to the past brings grief, and that has been my experience, exponentially multiplied as I circled back into the writing, the imagery, the progression, the old me.

Imagine what it was like to reread blog entries: I was walking, I traveled alone, I could get on a plane, I could go to Arizona, I could drag a twenty-two-inch suitcase behind me, I was still relatively mobile in spite of the fatigue of ALS. As I plumb past depths, the realization of both my blindness and my prescience washes over me in giant waves of incredulity. I was blind to just how far this thing was going to go, and yet I was clearly anticipating the losses, one by one, paper cut by paper cut, old normal into new normal. You can probably imagine the grief as I read about this person bemoaning his condition, even though he could walk and travel and work. And you can probably imagine the grief as I compared what he could do then to what I can do now.

Pictures are even worse.

As we put together a bike team to raise money for ALS Therapy Development Institute, a nonprofit ALS research group, my son Jon—who was building our website—innocently asked me for some biking pictures. Nothing I can think of ambushes me more than looking at pictures of Ev and me on a bike ride. It calls up all of the joy and fun and closeness of two people outdoors putting in the miles and letting life fall off onto the road. And I don't want to seem idealistic about the memory. There were times when we were both so tired, the headwind strong, the hills steep, the sun hot, or rain pelting that we just wanted to quit. But we learned to get through those times with a lot of encouragement: "You can do this, get on my wheel, and we'll do it together." My memories are about an equal partnership, overcoming physical and spiritual challenges. Flipping through pictures of both of us so fit, so physical, so happy in the privilege of riding together is an invitation to despair at what dis ease is doing.

Circling back is not for the faint of heart. Circling back is complex. It is hard to look at images from the past, frozen in their time, stripped of their context and feeling, and not judge them too harshly with the sharpened understanding of focused hindsight. I was doing the best I could at the time. You would do the same.

I now recognize that circling back is not really what I have been doing. Instead I have been spiraling down, deepening the experience so that what was once old normal confidence is now vulnerability, what was once an equal partnership riding on the roads must now be even more intimate in how we look out for each other. And in the ultimate spiral, as I flip through images of the effects of dis ease on my family and friends—and especially on my one true love, Ev—I must spiral into understanding that my fears were both well founded and inadequate in anticipation of what was to come.

When we are in the moment, it is easy to believe that we own a full understanding of the situation at hand. What I've come to realize is that as I move further and further into the experience of ALS, as my family and friends have their own interpretations and perceptions and epiphanies of these experiences, I am in a spiral of increasing awareness. What was then the complete package is now incomplete—requiring further analysis, further negotiation, and most importantly the humility to recognize the obvious.

I'm never going to fully get it.

We spend an inordinate amount of time trying to make sense of past failures and successes, attempting to control their effect on the future as if such control were attainable. In circling back, I spiraled down into the person I was, recently diagnosed— still walking and fearing the wheelchair, still breathing and fearing BiPAP, still speaking and fearing eye gaze technology. Spiraling down is all in, outside the lines, comforted by the futility of fear, embracing the contradiction of knowledge and ignorance in a miasma of fixing and working and looking and vulnerability and imagery old and new. And like delicate hammers striking disks of pure bronze in a space of melodic wonder, spiraling down is a balancing act on the edges of perfect harmony, in spite of my deafness.

That harmony was brought home to me recently with the birth of our first granddaughter, Hypatia. To say that I am over-the-top ecstatic, in love, sappy, dewy-eyed, wowed, totally into this tiny human being would be an understatement. And I am blown away by these feelings. Hypatia is the mirror in which I suddenly see the real projection.

She is, in my mind, perfection.

Before her daddy came into our lives, I wondered if I would have the emotional space for a son or daughter. Would I have enough love for his mother *and* him? He answered that question the minute he was born, and I realized that love's space had expanded, and there was more love to go around than I knew what to do with. When my second son was born, I suddenly realized that this loving space exponentially multiplies—no matter how many occupy its realm, there is always more love to give. When my sons introduced me to the women who are now their wives, that space opened up again, projecting out and underscoring what I had come to learn about love even to this day.

And now, this tiny beauty, who followed conversations back and forth at three days old, craning her neck when her daddy spoke, now taking her first solo steps before her first birthday, has completely stolen my heart, making me reconsider that man with ALS whose picture was taken in Millennium Park. Her birth was like the stars coming out at night, a realization of growth and sudden epiphany: that often the person we think we are is not reflected in the physical self we believe we project.

Her presence spirals down and down, transcending the dis ease that has framed my life these past four years.

I now look at the picture of the man in Millennium Park, and I realize he is waiting, waiting for something that will transform his outlook, reminding him that dis ease is more than ALS. I now look at the picture of that man, and I see love waiting to pour out on a tiny, helpless, long-awaited babe. I now look at the picture, and I don't see ALS at all. I just see me—heart open to the perfection and possibility of my beautiful Hypatia.

Suddenly, we are both on a spiral into joy and laughter and possibility beyond recognition.

22

FAITH, PART III
Wrestling with Angels

One of the most extraordinary things happened to Bruce on his fifty-eighth birthday. He received the gift of a lifetime, and he received it as he found himself wrestling with angels.

Intrigued? You should be.

First, about those angels.

The vivid metaphor of wrestling with angels is from the Bible. Depending on the interpretations, it's about Jacob's struggle with a man, an angel, or God. It can also be understood as Jacob confronting his failures, weaknesses, and sins, and facing God. In the biblical story, Jacob wrestles all night with an angel and is wounded, but then asks the angel for a blessing.

It was a request for a blessing that led to that extraordinary birthday for Bruce on March 1, 2014. Bruce and his family were at the Nobel Peace Prize Forum in Minneapolis to see the Dalai Lama. Bruce admires the holy man, and the 1998 Nobel Peace Prize winner was a keynote speaker at the event. I was the moderator of the question-and-answer session with His Holiness, and at its conclusion the Dalai Lama was asked, by an audience member, to bless those in attendance.

The holy man paused with a quizzical look on his face. "Blessing?" he replied. "Of course I'm Buddhist, so sometimes

I am a little bit skeptical of a so-called blessing. Blessing must come from our own action. Our own motivation."

His final comment drew sustained applause from the audience, and the session was supposed to end there. The Dalai Lama rose from his seat, but instead of walking to the nearby podium for an honorary presentation, he began walking toward the opposite end of the stage and pointing to where Bruce sat in the darkness.

"How would he know I was there?" Bruce recalled. "And then to point to me like, 'There you are! What are you doing over there?' Like he knew me all his life." To say Bruce was shocked would be a huge understatement.

In an unscripted moment, someone from the audience behind Bruce handed the Dalai Lama a white silk scarf with a colorful pattern on it. Holding it to his forehead, the Dalai Lama said, "Meanwhile, my blessing," and handed the scarf to a weeping Bruce.

Bruce wrestled with that moment for an entire week after the event and then realized His Holiness "didn't bless me at all. That's not what that was about. It was what he had talked about earlier. A blessing is in one's action and one's motivations and it's a charge. What blessings will you give? I have come to the conclusion that he was telling me that I'm not done, and that I'm not done until I'm finished."

The Bible doesn't say whether at any time in that dark night of wrestling with an angel Jacob thought that he was finished. He prevailed only to have the angel touch his hip, wounding it. But in the end, after asking for the angel's blessing and receiving it, Jacob became a man of faith.

In what, or where, or whom do you put your faith?

I'm talking about the kind of faith where there's a deep, emotionally involved kind of trust, one that is sacred. Many people will say they put their faith in God, Yahweh, Allah—a Supreme Power.

The dictionary also describes another kind of faith, which still relies on trust but in beliefs, in principles, in people, in religious traditions, in institutions, and in the self. Bruce is skeptical of the dichotomy. Instead, he wrestles with angels no matter what their source.

For me, faith begins in the human condition. We are born into these bodies, we live, and in the time we have been given, exacerbated by the lives we live, our bodies break down, and we die. The inexorable progression of death and birth is the beginning, and in that progression we are granted choices, real choices as to whether we shall be opened or closed to whatever world finds its way to our doorsteps. Choose to be open, and the circling gyre will open as well. Choose to be closed, and we collapse into flinty substance, angry and frustrated and lost.

For some, such statements of faith are the ultimate realism, humanism exponentially demonstrated by typical human functions. Such realism restricts our vision to that which can only be described scientifically, empirically, observable by the naked eye. But I do not mean these statements as such, for I do not fear the supernatural.

You see, for the past year I have been wrestling with angels.

Hard to believe, yet for the longest time, they have come to me in that space between sleep and wakefulness, when pain has suppressed my consciousness, disallowing unconsciousness to drift over me, in that space. In that pain came angels, and—like the Jacob I knew myself to be—I wrestled with them, embracing their presence, holding on to them for no reason other than the striving, the contest, to win or lose or draw in that pain. I wasn't even sure that they were real, but like Jacob, I had crossed the river of my dis ease to move into the promised life I knew was mine, and the fact that angels descended upon me in the night, wrestling with me—this frightened me into believing I might lose everything. ALS makes you think that way.

Like Jacob, I was not sure with whom I wrestled. At first, I thought they were supernaturals meant to taunt me with the visceral pain that they could inflict. Then I thought that perhaps they were those I had known from before, my grandparents, father-in-law, friends from this life but gone, transitioned into the next plane. Yet, it was not my beloveds gone before me. The more I tried to name the wrestlers, the more hidden my opponents' identities became. The more I tried to name my adversary, the more susceptible I became to the pain and hurt and fear.

I began to accept the fact that I was wrestling with the unknown. Wrestling with the unknown in the middle of the night wounded me, my own version of a dislocated hip, leaving me with a limp to the end of my days. But I have read the sacred texts, and I knew to be like Jacob, I could not let go until I was blessed—by pain and lost capacity and sadness. And I would hear myself speaking even though I was not conscious, "I cannot let you go until you have given your blessing to me."

In the blessing, I realized the unknown were angels.

I am sleeping better now. We have managed the pain that accompanies the full atrophy of muscles, the pulled threads of joints that lack movement and compression so that they ache and scrape, the neuropathic pain of edema in feet and hands. It is now rare that I wrestle angels in the middle of the night, and when I do, they are not the angels of pain and loss. Not in the middle of the night. Now, in that space between consciousness and sleep, between wakefulness and dreams, I know actual people, and I do not have to ask their blessing or wrestle from them my release. They wait patiently, kindly, ready for me and the day when I am ready for them.

But I still wrestle.

In the past two weeks, on dry land, on three different days, I have almost drowned. Through some combination of lifting and bracing and eating, my ability to breathe was compromised, leading to the most primal, prehistoric, adrenergic response a body can give. These are new angels, at once unknown to me, yet familiar as if we have wrestled before. They separate my mind from my body so that my mind remains calm yet amazed, watching as my body panics—fight or flight—pouring every chemical it can into the brink as if I am able-bodied and can run away or turn and fight. And of course, I cannot fight, nor can I run. And my response is one of great distress. I lie back just so, hoping the breath will come more easily, that my skin suddenly clammy with the shock of the oxygen deprivation will warm again, and the quiet center will return and bring me the peace I so desire.

Who are these angels with whom I wrestle now? In my distress, I cry aloud.

Now, I have a new secret name. I am Israel, for I have gazed upon the face of God, wrestled with her—not to win, not to lose, but to live as fully as I possibly can. And I have learned that wrestling with God is dis ease. In the sweat that pours off of me when I cannot breathe, the cellular fear that pours into me beyond all thinking, the full disruption of the calm, quiet, centered moment, is God. And God tells me do not accept this fear, this next symptom as anything but proof of my existence. And I say back, I will not go so gentle, and I will wrestle you until my nighttime is your morning.

And I am blessed.

There are remarkable angels in my life—my dearest love, my sons and their beautiful wives, my granddaughter, my very good friends, my caregivers who come for no reason but to reassure and love, even our two cats—and I have no problem reconciling who they are with the angels I have known. I do not awaken in the middle of the night so much anymore, my mind and body wrestling with the unknown. That was then, and this is now. But I am still ready to wrestle, to question, to proclaim that in the striving is life, wounded yet whole, ignorant yet wise. I now know that angels come from other places and no place at all. I now know that to be faithful, I must wrestle with God.

As a postscript, every once in a while our cats focus their gaze up above me, seeing something that I can only sense, raising the hairs on the back of my neck. And in their circling and grooming and play, I see angels. In those evening moments when Ev and I are finally alone together, I see angels. When I practice yoga, focusing inward and projecting my body outward, I see angels.

And when I occasionally awaken in the middle of the night, I sense them in the darkness, waiting still to be wrestled until I am wounded and blessed and finally taken home.

23

INSIDE OUT

Most of us face the world with well-worn armor, helmets pulled over our faces, ready to do battle. Others conceal with carefully crafted masks, wearing sadness like a heavy, musty velvet mantle. We humans tend to hide our real selves, wanting to protect the tender, soft, vulnerable parts of our essence. We project to the world the image we want to convey, not what is truly beneath the surface. There's risk in allowing people to see the "real" you—risk of rejection and ridicule.

We say and do the opposite of what we think and feel. In other words (as many therapists point out) our insides do not usually match our outsides. It is cause for many personal problems. It becomes more acute when dis ease is introduced—or rather, dis ease barges in and makes itself at home. Dis ease, in all its forms, strips one bare. There is nowhere to hide. All armor, all masks, all pretense is gone.

This condition is humanity at its most raw, its most vulnerable. It is frightening, but viewed in a different way, it is incredibly beautiful. What is left is the essence of self. The inside is the outside. And don't worry. You'll wear it well.

If there is anything that ALS teaches, it is that dis ease flips you on your ear and, not so ceremoniously, exposes your inside to the outside, burying any semblance of your old skin deep into your inner spaces. This isn't difficult to illustrate. While I probably shouldn't admit this, there is a picture of me that I love for its pure ego projection. Evelyn and I have just ridden our bikes 360 miles in six days—not Tour de France distances but certainly respectable. I am flexing my biceps as if I could ride forever, as if there is nothing to fear in my future, as if there will be no such thing as ALS.

The image is now buried deep in my psyche, and I only access it with great care or I will weep for its loss. When I look at that picture, I so easily become disconnected, discombobulated, a disarrayed example of humanity as I hold up the picture from the past against the person I am now. On a bad day, such easy perception is my dis ease.

I have never bought into Cartesian mind-body duality, so the overall effect of this gritty comparison is integrated—psychological, emotional, social, spiritual, physical, always physical. I suppose my friends in the counseling world might say that the effects are indicative of some form of depression. But this integrated effect is not depression. I think there is a better word, a better way to frame this holistic overarching ALS phenomenon. I prefer to think of it as diminished. In spite of all the mindful joy that I feel, the fact is that the physical overwhelms, playing a cruel trump card of diminishment.

If I play out the litany of loss, it is easy to conclude that I have been diminished. This body no longer moves with any purpose except to occupy space. My breath moves at a capacity that is less and less able to sustain my body. My voice is weakened to the point where others cannot hear me—no breath, muscle weakness, and spasms in the face and neck. My hands are atrophied with curling fingers and opposite thumbs, one flexed and one extended. My temperature is perpetually on the cold side with hands that are like ice and feet that swell in pain yet bungee jump between too hot and too cold. My mouth, tongue, and throat tire easily and eating leaves me out of breath. Connect the litany of loss with that earlier picture of health—the diminished person seems like the only way to reconcile the two images.

But there are other ways to seek reconciliation. My life before ALS was carefully planned, a litany of future projection.

At home, I planned to sleep in the arms of my one true love, to be awake, so very awake to her presence in my life. I planned to be there for my boys and their true loves and the children that they would have. I planned to cook for birthdays and anniversaries, at Thanksgiving and Christmas, during three-day weekends and one-night chili cook-offs, on holidays and holy days. I planned to be the husband and father and grandfather of legend. Professionally, I planned to bring a rational voice and compassionate love to the education of children, the emotional healing humanity requires, the design of systems that would support people, not chew them up. I planned to be the best friend anyone could ever have. I planned to make beautiful music. Before ALS, I could see my plans opening into limitless vistas.

Now, I am cured of planning. Now, I pay attention to the losing—hand dexterity, back strength, neck strength, swallowing, breathing, vocal presence—all joining the legs and arms and torso already gone. And with the losses, I have struggled to play catch-up and turn the old ways into new ways, which I now realize are just barely ahead as the losses pile up behind.

And yet, maybe I am not cured. I still have plans—final words, time spent, memories, music.

I plan to end in a better space, always a better space.

If I have learned anything from ALS, it is that being turned on your ear is not a singular event. With patience, all things turn, and turn again. There is no big announcement, no one thing that rotates me away from feeling sorry for myself toward that person I want to be. In spite of my whining, I work hard for spaces devoid of soul-killing feelings—deep resentment, crushing bitterness, prolonged anger. It isn't that I don't own major reserves of these feelings, but grim feelings have no payoff; they depress colors, muffle sounds, numb the touch, and leave me hopeless in dis ease. So I do my best to acknowledge them, communicate them, concentrating instead on things that bring me back into the here-and-now space, where the beauty of living is so much clearer, even if it feels shortened by circumstance.

There is another way to see the space.

My friend and teacher Matt loves the visual arts. They speak to him intellectually in the same way that music speaks to me. Multidimensional, existent on many levels, planes of seeming conflict ultimately colliding into harmony. When Matt talks about art, it is as if the universe has tapped a secret message in a code with which I can barely keep up. Often, it isn't so much his analysis of any given artwork but his passion and insight that move me. This experience parallels my own discovery, intellectual insight, spiritual awakening in dis ease and its clarion ALS. Recently, in commenting on a work by Matisse, he noted how we tend to see our inner space and our external perceptions as disconnected, even on different planes. Yet, as he gazed at a painting, he perceived just how the artist connected mind with body, and he cried in the epiphany.

Matt maintains that inner space is neutral—a source of strength and resilience. He says the inner is what we breathe into, the hum we experience when all around us is silence. He believes this space is the metaphysical place where we experience heartbreak and ache and loneliness, joy, and wonder. Inner space precedes objective perception.

We share these experiences from time to time, Matt and I, in spite of the fact that we occupy different space. As he shares his experience of Matisse, I cannot help but let his words connect to my inner space. I look inside as if a window has been opened, not by the artist but by the realization in his words. As my friend posits the difficulty in perceiving each other's inner space—in fully understanding each other's inner source of strength—I realize that this is truth, yet it is not my experience at all. Had we spoken on the topic four years ago, I would have intellectually nodded, agreeing with his analysis. But of course, that was then, and now things are very different.

Listen! ALS has turned me inside out, my innermost vulnerabilities and secrets worn as an outer skin for everyone to see, the strong and confident vitality of flexed muscles pushed inward into spaces that only I know. Suddenly, as my friend speaks, I am connected. My inner spaces are pushed out wherever I am, and compassion and understanding and unity in the human condition pour out and over my heart. ALS only overwhelms my body. My soul still sings, now for all to hear. My spirit breathes, revealed as my skin is pushed inside. The picture I so carefully access is now a negative reversal of the person I am.

I still flex my muscles, inside and out, ready with a new plan, diminished but stronger and more resilient than any picture can be.

24

DIS EASE YOGA

Those who practice yoga say it is life changing. Those of us who are as flexible as a piece of lumber are not so sure. I admire yoga's rich history, more than five thousand years old, but I run into a few mental roadblocks in understanding concepts like grounding and spinal energy. In fact, I was sitting in my slumped-over and crooked version of the lotus position during a special yoga class taught by Bruce's mentor Matthew Sanford, when Matthew said to a student, "Breathe into your spine for God's sake!" I had no idea what that meant. The student understood though, and he made proper adjustments. What was remarkable was that both teacher and student were in wheelchairs.

I was in the Monday assistive-yoga class that Bruce takes with Matthew and a room full of people with various physical challenges, along with a small army of able-bodied assistants. A couple of months before, Bruce mentioned he was taking a yoga class. I must have had a surprised/skeptical/bemused look on my face because I couldn't understand how a person in a wheelchair could be doing yoga. Bruce invited me to attend a class, and what I saw opened my eyes. It was beautiful to watch the students and Matthew work together. Bruce would say his life with ALS has been transformed because of yoga and his deep friendship with his teacher and mentor.

Matthew's own story is a remarkable one. At the age of thirteen he was paralyzed from the chest down in a horrible car crash that killed his father and sister. His doctors encouraged him to leave his old body behind and concentrate on overcoming his disability. Matthew had other ideas and began studying yoga and other bodywork. He is the founder of a Minnesota-based nonprofit that teaches both those with disabilities and those who are able-bodied how to move, breathe, and balance.

What is very clear is that while Bruce continues to lose physical capacity, he is also gaining life energy and a freedom that transcends his failing body. Often when we meet, Bruce has his fancy stereo system on at a volume that can shake the walls. His taste in music is wonderfully vast, and I have heard music with Bruce I've never listened to before. There was a song by the Avett Brothers playing one afternoon: "There's a darkness upon me that's flooded in light."

Bruce, despite the darkness of ALS, really is cloaked in light and love. Yoga allows him to feel the space beyond his wheelchair, and it's a space that has allowed for amazing spiritual growth.

You can see it.

It is probably indicative of my old normal before ALS that I honestly regarded yoga as an activity for my wife, not for a weight-lifting, biking, swimming, semi-running fifty-something-year-old male who believed he was going to live forever. I thought it was nice for the YMCA to offer yoga, even though I secretly thought their main focus ought to be on weight lifting and crushing physical fitness. I believed that yoga was for other people, especially those who might not understand the inner peace of weight lifting, biking, swimming, and running. I never in a million years thought that I would practice yoga. It took a diagnosis of ALS and an awakening to the phenomenon of dis ease for me to reconsider.

For nearly two years, I have held words and thoughts and symbols and sighs in my heart concerning my practice of yoga. I know the idea that a person with ALS can practice yoga—unable to control any physical function, totally reliant on the goodwill and expertise of volunteers and loved ones—might spawn incredulity. I might have seen it the same way two years ago. But the yoga story that I carry is one that has given me deep gifts, both tangible and intangible. I want to share some of those gifts, not because I believe everyone should become a yogi—a student of yoga—but rather that in this particular experience is the complexity of human dis ease and what it means to have ALS. And in addition, yoga has also shown me what it means to excavate my spirit until ideas of success and failure, growth and regression, consciousness and unconsciousness, awareness and awakening are turned on their ear.

So on the day after Thanksgiving in 2012, almost two years from diagnosis and with the encouragement of friends and family, I started adaptive yoga. Adaptive yoga allows a person with disability to find centeredness through restorative and strengthening poses and breathing, always breathing. During each class the darkness lifts from me for a few moments, my sense of breath increases, the compacted feeling that comes from progressive physical loss and overreliance on mechanical wonders such as power chairs lightens, and I reach out beyond my confinement. Now, though I find myself conscious of another loss and another each week, I am also aware of divinity—each of us communing through some variation of Holy Spirit in breath and pose and selfless friends and teachers lifting us into divine spaces. Invariably, joy and tears combine for me each session.

Preparing for yoga is no small task, and as ALS has progressed, it has become more and more complicated. Our ability as students with disability to find our way into practice is more or less dependent on the goodness of others. At the very least, someone helps us into the classroom. And most of us need help with dressing and help with feeding; some like myself need help with breathing. We require assistance so that our equipment is ready to go. And getting into our transportation, getting out of our transportation, getting into and out of buildings can be complicated. Each of us has our own private challenge just to be present in the yoga classroom.

When I tell people about my practice, I am often met with

disbelief. How can you practice yoga when you can't move your arms or your legs, when your breathing continues to decline? My acquaintances and friends, usually able-bodied and possibly stuck in their own frames of reference, tend to be incredulous—or they react as if adaptive yoga is cute, somehow diminished, not a real yoga practice. But the reality is that just as God is not in the clouds, yoga is not in the pose. It resides in the base and the space we create—our bodies, ourselves, our community, our discipline.

And our practice is as real and tangible as the disabilities each of us carries.

Like most people who come to yoga, I have found in the practice a negotiation between mind and body, what I think and what I can do, and the energy that binds them together. But in that negotiation—mind, body, and energy—is the opportunity to experience spirit and wisdom emergent from the mind-body dialogue. Mind, body, spirit, energy, wisdom, all interact and intertwine, striving for conscious and unconscious attention.

Yoga is also the space where my insecurities arise, asking questions like, why are you wasting the time of these good people with a body that can do nothing without their significant support? And yoga is the space where answers emerge from the discipline: Accept the body that you have; thank it for what it is and what it can do. Accept the creative love of the volunteers and teachers in this room. Practice yoga.

I have attended yoga as often as possible, on Monday evenings with either Ev or my kids, and on Friday with good friends—yogis in their own right—who very generously donate their time and physical strength to support my practice. Often, my teachers will drop in to my home and practice with me. The classes school me in understanding the ways my new body works. Great attention is paid to the smallest detail in the spine, the diaphragm, the energy of breath as it flows from grounded space through my limbs, head, and heart. Each of us—those with traumatic injury, cerebral palsy, MS, chronic pain, and even me with ALS—finds our own way into the knowledge and practice our teachers present.

The concentrated focus on spinal energy for a person with ALS—a person who one would assume has lost spinal awareness—reveals vast spaces for spiritual growth in spite of the physical loss. The students who so graciously allow me to join them are remarkable in their physical progress. Some show new capability, and in their joyful growth, I must remember that even though ALS robs me of the ability to gain strength from physical activity, my practice of a yogic routine has enormous energetic, emotional, spiritual benefit. And of course, I receive definite physical benefit in moving a body confined by paralysis. Each class is different, neither better nor worse but complementary one to the other.

After each class, I am exhausted yet more aligned in space than before I began, more alive to the spirit in the breath, more engaged with the beauty of human-to-human contact. I mark epiphanies exploding into my awareness or creeping quietly into the edges of consciousness. Each class requires physical engagement, more than was ever required of me when I was able-bodied. The philosophy of my teachers is to illuminate human understanding through the more readily discernible physical acts of yoga. Meanwhile, they challenge us to find deep meaning in the discovery of the transience and uniqueness that each of us brings to the practice. And strangely, my soul is engaged. No wonder I am so tired at the end.

During any given class, at any given time, I can expect that the practice will remove my carefully constructed facade, layer by layer, piece by piece, until my dis ease is fully exposed.

Yoga requires total honesty. At times, I enter the room, and the new challenges presented by my body make the immediacy of practice all but unrecognizable. Yesterday I could hold up my hand, today I require the assistance of loving volunteers. Yesterday I could find space between my pelvis and my shoulder, today I slump and compress into my lower back. Yesterday I could sit up straight and tall, today my wheelchair provides the only straightness available. It is not uncommon for me to focus on some small physical requirement, one that I could do even one week ago, and recognize that it is now impossible without the aid of another—and I grieve that loss in momentary gulps of re-alization and sorrow that pass through me like saltwater tears. I cannot help it, marking the losses week to week.

Yet, I can still remember the energetic feel of pressing down to lift up, of expanding inward the lower ribs to expand outward through my shoulders. Our practice of yoga truthfully embraces the physical loss for which we weep and the energetic lift that we celebrate, yet our minds will always bring a sense of infancy to the practice. Even if we did not have disabilities, normal aging would dictate that as we gain understanding, we also lose physi-cal capacity.

Our minds are amazed by such phenomena.

We can interpret our amazement as loss from the progres-sion of disease, or we can be amazed by our rebirth into a new existence. The body doesn't lie. It tells us to be the persons that we are, to calm the mind in the practice that can be accomplished today, and to be grateful for the discipline. It is the mind that panics, judges, chooses anxiety over serenity.

It would be dishonest to deny the grief that accompanies the losses I have marked in my practice. My son and daughter-in-law, my friends, my teachers all grieve with me. The discipline re-quires the honesty to face such feelings, and yet this is not where we choose to live. We face the thought together, calmly note that it exists, and we move back into the practice. But this is hard for me, for I have always been taught that to give is the best blessing, and it is difficult to perceive just what I am giving in my highly assisted practice.

Then I remember what I have learned—to receive is the gift. Yoga is just an avenue to deeper insight, an expansion of breath against the restriction of some perceived elastic band around my torso, an opening of heart against fear of awareness. Awakening to such psychic, spiritual, emotional, faith-filled space holds at bay the panic hidden in the physical loss. It is as if I am on the circling gyre, simultaneously spiraling up and down in opposite directions—one spiritual, climbing into the rarefied awareness, and one physical, falling into deep velvet loss.

I do not know how long I will be able to continue. I hope

until I die. My physical capacity continues to wane, and the logistics of attendance are more and more complicated. Each week is an intertwining of grief and joy, and that seems to me correct. I am encouraged in ways you might find fantastical. Last Monday, I decided, would be my last Monday evening. The logistics are just so difficult. But then, I received a note from the son of my friend Paul, telling me how much he missed his dad in the year since his father died. And at yoga that evening, after centering, I required my BiPAP just to breathe easily, just like Paul when he practiced. And I felt his presence surrounding me with encouragement, and I knew that it wasn't quite time. I still have time and practice and discipline.

ALS requires it, dis ease insists upon it, and so yoga balances tears and laughter, realization and unawareness, the spiral up and the spiral down, each week, the discipline and the practice.

25

FAITH, PART IV
What's Love Got to Do with It?

Kids who grew up in the 1940s, '50s, and '60s were not likely to hear the words "I love you" from their parents. Fathers of the time might have offered awkward hugs on occasion, but demonstrative displays of emotion were the exception, not the rule.

Fritz Wurzer was one of those fathers.

He came from stoic German stock. He signed birthday cards "Love, Dad," but I can't recall him saying, "I love you." The closest he would come was to say, "Me too" if you were to utter those precious words to him. I write this with no anger, only love. I know without a doubt my father loved his family.

Once it became clear that the lymphoma in my dad's spleen had turned deadly and his kidneys were shutting down, I had the great gift of talking with him in the hospital on the final day he had his eyes open and was present and attentive. He never spoke during that time. His dementia affected his speech. He was mostly mute, which was ironic, given that he had been a teacher and had taken great pleasure in lecturing.

Holding his hand—and between torrents of tears—I thanked him for all that he had done for me and for our family, and told him how very much he would be missed. I told him that I thought he was an amazing man, which elicited a surprised raise of his eyebrows and a bemused little smile. He was indeed amazing for how he lived, as gracefully as possible, with all the insults that dementia and other disease had heaped on him. Finally, I told him that I loved him, and I kept telling him that, in various ways, during his last days. As he took his final few breaths, I hope love was the last of his memories to die.

At Palm Sunday services a little more than a month after my father died, I sat in the front pew of the Good Samaritan United Methodist Church in Edina, Minnesota—Bruce's church—and waited to hear Bruce give a special sermon. The prayer preceding the sermon had me in tears.

> Holy and compassionate God, this day began with the bright sounds of praise to you, yet too soon when life is hard, like the disciples we run away. We are afraid of loving as you have loved us. Forgive us with your deep and wide mercy; make us brave to walk with you even in the darkness, trusting you will bring us from fearful living into the hope and light of your deep and abiding love.

Once Bruce finished his sermon, titled "From the Silence," the rest of the congregation was crying too. Here is the sermon, as delivered by Bruce on that Palm Sunday.

Claire and Matt sit in a small office in the neurological wing at the clinic. The clinician has come to get me, just finishing up my own quarterly clinic visit, to ask if I would consider meeting them. I am so fatigued, but as she tells me that Matt is in his last weeks with ALS, that they read my blog, find my words helpful, and would like to meet, the only human choice is yes. I roll in, my daughter-in-law driving my chair, the clinician at my side. We immediately feel the desperate, resigned love, five people shaped by ALS in this moment together. Matt speaks through an iPad application, "I'm doing as well as I can." Claire sits slightly behind him, her hands on his shoulders willing him not to slip away just yet. She holds it together through some superhuman effort, telling us that she had to take Matt to the hospital, and with a Do Not Intubate order, hospital staff were afraid they couldn't bring him around. A chaplain had been summoned to pray over him, and for some reason, when the chaplain touched Matt's hand, his eyes opened, he sat up and immediately started breathing again. Her tears belie her attempt at humor, "I have to find that chaplain to thank him, but I want him there the next time." The next time looms over all of us in the room. "I am just not ready to let him go. Our kids are young, and when we went to the hospital, the oldest asked if his daddy was going to die tonight. I am just not ready."

ALS crams a lot of story into short, breathless nights, minutes and hours and days and weeks of passion story.

Today is Palm/Passion Sunday. We Methodists tend to cram a lot of story into this day, partly because we don't like to dwell too much on how dark the week feels, partly because we are so busy with lives that seem beyond the pale of such a story. If we could, we would probably compress the passion story even more, something along the lines of a tweet:

> Jesus—triumph, Temple, Passover; Gethsemane—prayer, despair, arrest, denial; Pilate—Herod, trial; Golgotha— cross, cry, acceptance, death.

We Methodists cram a lot of story into this one Sunday.

In spite of its darkness, I have always loved holy week. It is the complete package, a story where each of us can find some element to which we can relate. Each of us knows what it means to succeed, perhaps even triumph. Each of us knows how passing such success can be, like turning a corner into sunlight only to become aware of the next storm on the horizon. Many of us have learned that success is nothing more than the question, What have you done for me lately? Indeed in my old life, no success was ever good enough because I knew that waiting just beyond the triumph—if I did not immediately move to address it—was possible and imminent disaster. Who among us has never felt betrayed or denied by friends or lovers, those we thought we could count on the most? Who among us has not perceived, even just a little bit, the lie that we are in control? Who among us has never felt so alone that we are sure even God has turned away? This is the stuff of life, blistering our emotional overlay into thick yet well-worn calluses of experience. Each of us knows how it feels to be helpless in the face of events. Each of us can point to some event where we feel like we have been figuratively, if not literally, crucified.

And each of us can understand viscerally, primally, the question, Why have you forsaken me?

You see how human the story is, this holy week? Jesus in the garden asking God to take the cup away. And here is something I believe. If he has become the human the Scriptures tell us, then he would not have said, "I will drink if this is your will." Humans don't start with acceptance, with "if it be thy will." We have to hear the nothing voice on the edges of a cold wind, wrestle with God's silence, balance in ever-increasing despair and frustration between anger and sadness at the perceived lack of response. Jesus was alone in his loneliness, facing his own mortality, his own dis ease, just as we are alone in our loneliness facing our own dis ease, our own crucifixions. Christ's loneliness screams betrayal and denial and anticipated pain. His loneliness breathes total despair. In his loneliness is his overwhelming humanity, longing to hear his father answer, entreating his father to break his heartbreaking silence. The cup of mortality will not be taken from Jesus, for now he is one of us, and mortality is our human gift.

"Will no one stay awake with me?"

When I was first diagnosed, I composed my own variations on the theme of "Take this cup from me." The more I learned about what was coming, the more frightened and angry I became. What disease could possibly steal more completely the life that I loved than ALS? To be stripped so naked of all the things I enjoyed—to hug, to sing, to kiss, to eat, to ride, to speak, to travel, to breathe—the cruelty was beyond my comprehension, and I could see a future where every loss would be another opportunity for anger and fear, slashing livid red streaks across my vision and into the very core of my being. No one could understand this, no one. And I would be alone. I cried aloud to God, and I swear to you God did not answer.

I was so afraid.

Three and a half years ago, and dis ease has brought me to the precipice: Will I live into the life I have been given, or die in anger, frustration, grief? I don't hear any answers from God, at least I didn't at first. But then something happens. The answers appear, not as I saw them but in their own guise: first in a trickle of prayers and "I love you's" and quiet solace as I begin to tell people, "I have ALS, we have ALS." Then the torrent opens. My brother tells me I can lick this, I can fight it. I want to argue, but then I realize this isn't about me, it is about him. ALS has opened him to examining his own life, how he would react, what seems true to him—my disease and his mortality molded into deep reflection.

I don't argue with him, I listen and open a little bit.

A healer calls me and says, "You are angry, hurt by your body. You must forgive yourself, forgive your body; it is only doing what it is meant to do. If you do not forgive yourself . . ." She leaves the thought unfinished, allowing my imagination, my creativity to build around it.

I don't argue with her, I listen and open a little bit more.

I have to tell my colleagues, the college that I lead. I have to admit my mortality and vulnerability and weakness and fatigue. I had invited them to believe that no burden would ever be too much for me, that I am strong enough to carry any load required. I must now lose that narrative and admit my humanity, and I am scared, for I know that sharks circle at the smell of blood. I write them a letter. I tell them I love working on their behalf, being their dean, that I want to continue until I cannot. And then I write the vulnerability: "If I cannot do the job, I will step down." Like cascades of water pouring out on a desiccated soul, they respond—notes and office stop-ins and meetings in the hall— love and support that could not have been written better into a Hollywood movie script.

Their love opens me even more.

I have to tell the choir—a group for which I still carry twinges of regret, even a little guilt, for stepping away from them to become dean of the college. Our pastor brings Evelyn and me into the room, and we tell our new story, and the choir listens, quiet, respectful, eyes on us and looking away. And then they stand and surround us and cry and touch and pray over us so that the only thing we can feel is love, pure love. A year later on an Easter Sunday, in a "Hallelujah Chorus" that I can no longer climb the steps to sing, they will leave the choir loft and surround us again, lifting our voices with their strength.

What wondrous love is this.

Six weeks ago, I attended a lecture with His Holiness the Dalai Lama. At the end of the question-and-answer period, he was asked to bless over 3,300 people in attendance. His answer was that he was skeptical about blessing, that blessing comes through our own individual action and motivation. It was a beautiful answer—through our actions we perpetuate blessing on and on and on, rather than waiting for blessing to happen. When the program ended, he suddenly turned toward me, walked across the stage to me, held a scarf hastily given to him up to his forehead and said, "Meanwhile, my blessing . . ." And he handed me the scarf. For a week I struggled in confusion as people asked me, "What was it like to be blessed by the Dalai Lama?" I tried to describe it, but I knew my frame of reference was wrong. And then it dawned on me. It wasn't about a singular blessing, him to me. It was a charge for intentional action. It was another awakening to open even more to the love that is all around us. Not, "Meanwhile my blessing," finished and done. Instead, "Meanwhile, my blessing . . ." Unfinished, a call to us to embrace love—for love's action and motivation and intent can and must be lived into, breathed into until you cannot breathe any longer.

The opposite of love is not hate; it is fear.

The greatest challenge of dis ease is that the moment fear overwhelms you, the moment you are dragged into your own soul-wrenching vulnerability, this is precisely the moment to open yourself to love. It is fear that causes us to feel estranged and alone, apart from God and from each other. To be closed off from love is crushing, angry loneliness, whether intentional or not. To be closed is to think that God only speaks with a voice—

words and sentences and phrases and paragraphs. To be closed is to be sick with the reality that impending death presents.

To be open is to embrace your own great big messy humanity, to cry in sadness but not despair, to recognize presence in the emptiness of the bitter moment of truth, to be afraid but not fearful. Dis ease presents the choice of being open or closed, and opening to her lessons, her gifts, her challenges, is not easy. But dis ease clarifies vision, bringing sight to the blindness of what you thought you knew about living, light to the darkness of cynicism that life's grief piled upon itself can foster. I know ALS is a horror, yet when fully embraced, it has taught me, it has revealed to me pure unsullied, uncontaminated, unbelievable love.

In my heart of hearts, I know that love never dies.

We sit together in a small room in the neurological wing at the clinic. What can anyone possibly say in such a holy moment? Matt's eyes implore me to tell what I know. I hear myself, words from another place, wrestled from angels in long and winding dialogues between sleep and wakefulness, "You will never be alone, Claire, for Matt's love will survive this physical shell of the body. You know this is true. Close your eyes, and think of how much he loves you and how much you love him. That love will always be with you. Your children will know him for his love and his bravery and his courage. And they will know his love through you. There will be sadness, at first overwhelming, but as all of you move together with that love that you have known, that sadness will become beautiful, a source of strength, a place that you can visit and be made whole again." We cry, Claire and Matt and the clinician and me and my daughter-in-law. We cry together at this most holy and human and loving moment, and out of our blessed silence I begin to understand the acceptance.

"God, into your hands I commend my spirit."

26

WE KNOW HOW THIS ENDS

Bruce is living—gloriously and fully, living as only one who knows his days are measured can live—with grace, great love, and sorrow over what is to come.

The end of our time together is drawing close. I can feel it but don't want to say that out loud. It's childish to think that not talking about dying will somehow stave off the inevitable.

We know how this ends.

That knowledge tethered me to primal fears and petty worries, and had I given in to them, I would have missed the opportunity to bear witness to the brilliant conclusion of a life that in many ways reflected my own. I just didn't understand the possibilities in the beginning.

A friend asked why I kept our series of radio conversations going over several years when, as Bruce was slowly dying, so were both my marriage and my father. All were nearing their separate ends, with both my dad and my marriage declared dead within a day of each other. My friend acknowledged that it seemed such pain would have been too much for her to bear. I wish I had an insightful answer as to why—despite soul-piercing grief—I kept going to Bruce's house and starting our conversations with "How's your heart?" when mine was breaking. On one level, Bruce's progression mirrored my father's. And while my father wasn't able to voice his feelings, Bruce was. In essence, Bruce became my father's voice, and I learned how to connect with him thanks to Bruce's sage advice. On a much more profound level, Bruce taught me how to transform pain into something more powerful. In the past, I would try to deflect, deny, or drown out my various forms of dis ease. This confluence of events wasn't going to make that possible. I was going to have to go through the fire instead of skirting it, or worse, cowering and trying to hide from the preordained conclusion.

We know how this ends.

It will end in tears and sadness. It must. To know such a remarkable spirit with so much compassion, wisdom, and love is a once-in-a-lifetime gift. To have that spirit leave is heartbreaking, even though the leave-taking is necessary. Many were touched by a man whose body could not be healed, but who tried in his final days to heal his fellow humanity.

We know how this ends.

It might have ended sooner.

Bruce has long talked about "winding down" and what he was seeing, in long reveries where he'd contemplate his life and what's to come. In "Love Notes from the Universe," a blog entry from December 2013, he wrote:

> Less than two months ago, I truly believed that my time was finished. I was always tired, and I spoke in whispers, afraid that if my voice was any louder, it would overwhelm the holy act of dying. I planned my funeral, mustered all the energy I could find for one final push of writing, reframed my dis ease in the comfort of a life well-lived and the regret of a life cut short before its time. I was convinced this would be my last Christmas, my last anniversary, the winding down with the family and friends that I love. In that time, my heart became very quiet, and my hearing acute. Suddenly I realized that whether on the stage in front of a thousand people or in the quiet intimacy of my own thoughts, the love notes that before had to disrupt my awareness in order for me to perceive them, required no such violence. In the quiet solitude of winding down is the ocean roar of love.

That is the one great lesson Bruce Kramer, master teacher, has tried to instill in word and action. Life is love. Love with an open heart and the realization that we all are meant to love and be loved. It is our birthright. Each one of us.

We know how this ends. It ends with sadness that is achingly beautiful and pure love for a life lived full and well.

When we have done all the work we were sent to do, we are allowed to shed our body, which imprisons our soul like a cocoon encloses the future butterfly.
                                        —Elisabeth Kübler-Ross

We know how this ends.

Lines from William Butler Yeats's "Sailing to Byzantium" reverberate in my soul, so that I cannot think of phrases more expressive than his. This "is no country for old men." I can think of all kinds of reasons why, none of which seems particularly credible. Perhaps it is recurrent respiratory infections, nothing much on their own but one after the other, iterations and variations on a theme of exhaustion through conditions that are hard to shake. Perhaps it is the anticipation, even in the autumn, of the deep freeze of late January and early February in the frozen North, when on a day when the temperature reaches the teens, good Minnesotans shed their clothes down to shirtsleeves and enjoy the balmy weather even though it is colder than sin. Maybe it is the cold summer whispering to me, in Yeats's words, "Soul clap its hands and sing, and louder sing," of subjects I can barely understand, let alone perceive. Or perhaps it is a new phase in the inexorable song of dis ease—a new beginning as I wind down to the inevitable. Illness, winter, summer, dis ease's song, one is not mutually exclusive of the other, but the energy that each requires, compared to the energy that I possess, puts me in the deficit.

I am almost always at least a little bit tired.

This is new territory, a new geography where living seems noisy, and I feel quiet, where two or three hours of napping on top of a good night of sleep is normal, where I am happy to just sit and think, to doze and listen to music wending its way in and out of consciousness. It is a space where the definition of living remains constant, but the meaning shifts and mewls—horizontal to vertical, cries to calls, life to laughter. It isn't that I am not awake, alive to possibility. It's simply that projecting outward seems less and less relevant, whereas aligning energy—above and behind, head and heart, body and soul—is a far better use of life force. And even though I occupy new space, there is still a consistency that I recognize as self.

I still love. I still feel. I still desire. I still recognize possibility.

ALS has its own gravity, strong enough that each repeated orbit is always just a bit smaller, a hair closer to its sun, a flick of the wrist of the master fisherman reeling me in until I am caught and netted. That ALS affords any orbit at all is a marvel, for its main effects are an exaggeration of the laws of physics that keep all of us firmly grounded on the earth. As I spiral down, my perception is blurred so that I cannot tell whether the weight I feel is due to ALS's great mass—so vast that light does not escape its pull, and so hot that purification by its fire is all one can expect from the encounter. With the completion of each orbit, my existence becomes more and more about being, less and less about doing, and the silence of the space roars its presence.

In this space, verbal expression seems so inadequate, words less meaningful. I find myself turning to music, to the "sages standing in God's holy fire," naming the feelings, the experiences, the Godhead of my dis ease, the "singing-masters of my soul." More harmonic than tonal, more fundamental than overtone, more rhythmic than steady beat, it is music that defines the emotion: the sunshine and brightness of E major; the steady and assured F fundamental; B-flat minor, a sadness that hangs five times from the staff like crows on a wire. Words fulfill their meaning through phrases molding and shaping the line, so that its apex hangs in the speck of time that defines temporal existence. And as with all orbits there is a point of no return, for it is only a matter of time before I will be consumed by heat and friction and cool atmosphere returning this body to the constant motion of rest and essence. I am assured and reassured by my faith in what I hear and experience.

"An aged man is but a paltry thing," yet I am thankful.

I am thankful for a family as loving and supportive as mine. I am thankful for the communities that have held out their arms and embraced me with love and tears and straightened fingers and blankets and peanut butter and music and the space to fall asleep.

I am thankful for the opportunity to get to know great people in the medical field, compassionate men and women who walk beside me and heroically seek respite for me. And as strange as it may seem, I am thankful for a life framed by true love and ALS allowing me to grow beyond the lesser person I could have been. When I consider the person I might have become—blind and ignorant and tone deaf in a world of art and knowledge and music—the gifts bestowed by Evelyn, my one true love, and my teacher ALS are beyond comprehension.

I know how this sounds. It sounds like I am resigning my-self to death, even though the silence from which I write feels very much alive. But if I am resigned, then like everything else I have experienced through ALS, it is much better to be ready, to anticipate rather than pretend that life remains constant. Like preparation for the performance of a beautiful yet challenging piece of music, this quiet serves as rehearsal time, a human at-tempt in the great liturgy that frames life to try to get it right. Perhaps in this final performance, I am finally granted the gift of singing "of what is past, or passing, or to come."

Now, my loves and I are allowed to practice for the moment when silence is the best gift, in spite of the noise that must al-ways frame the ending. It allows me conservation of energy and liberation of spirit as I spend time, delicious and beautiful, with friends. It allows me to breathe in the honeyed sweetness, the life presence of my one true love, unencumbered by the baggage we think we will require, supported by the truths we will actually need—love and life and laughter and tears.

All of us will know the "artifice of eternity."

In the years since ALS framed my life, I have sought to be

engaged fully with life as I knew it. Now, it seems more important to engage with life as it is. I hope this means more time with
loved ones, both friends and family; more evenings with Ev listening to the local classical station, drinking in each other's presence and knowing full well it will never be enough; more yoga
with Jon and Kirsten; more time with David carefully shaving
me, loving joyful visits with Hypatia and Athena, family meals
where I can barely keep up with the conversation; more naps
during the day and deep sleep at night. I hope this means more
time to think, to listen, to perceive that in the silence is life and
death and life again.

And maybe, dis ease will grant me the gift of a song bestowed, that my loves might carry our music into the great
unknown.

ACKNOWLEDGMENTS

Writing is often romanticized as a singular and lonely act, but in our case nothing could be further from the truth. We are grateful for the support and inspiration of so many who helped us in this project.

We first acknowledge Bruce's family, generous with encouragement, critique, and most important the understanding that writing with a disease like ALS creates its own challenges that require enormous support in order for the writing to take place. You read about these remarkable people in this book; know that it would not have been possible to write without them.

We recognize Minnesota Public Radio, which courageously provided a platform to tell a story as it truly exists rather than as a feel-good kicker narrative glamorized into something that it is not. Minnesota Public Radio stood with Cathy as she found her way into the story and remains supportive as the story comes to its natural ending. We especially thank Cathy's producer at Minnesota Public Radio, Jim Bickal, who edited the MPR stories with great sensitivity.

Bruce deeply appreciates the support of his wonderful volunteer care network. These people sat silently and listened to him dictate; adjusted his fingers, his body, and his feet; fed him potato chips; offered moral support; watched over him as he slept; and talked with him when he needed to talk. Each one of these wonderful volunteers is an angel on earth.

We acknowledge the vast number of people who engaged with us on social media with encouragement and suggestions as we sought to turn this story into something useful and worthy. One person we call out in particular is Tom Vandervoort, who got us together at the beginning.

Cathy recognizes the care her father received from his wonderful caregivers and her mother. Caregiving for anyone with a terminal disease requires change and growth, and her father's experience illuminated the beauty of the care he received.

We thank our editor at the University of Minnesota Press, Erik Anderson. His kindness, sensitivity, tough love, and commitment to this book inspired us and encouraged us to write beyond ourselves. We cannot thank him enough.

Finally, we are grateful to each other for the opportunity to work together. Writing a book could take a friendship and dash it on the rocks of life. We are happy to report that this was not our experience, and the project of writing together has deepened our friendship.

BRUCE H. KRAMER is former Dean of the College of
Education, Leadership, and Counseling at the University of St.
Thomas in the Twin Cities. Prior to his long tenure in higher
education, he was a high school principal in Bangkok, Cairo,
and Stavanger, Norway. He is coauthor of *Leading Ethically in
Schools and Other Organizations* and wrote Dis Ease Diary, a
popular blog about living with ALS.

CATHY WURZER is host of *Morning Edition* for Minnesota
Public Radio News and cohost of *Almanac,* a weekly public
affairs program on Twin Cities Public Television. In 2011 she
began talking with Bruce Kramer about his experience with
ALS in a series on *Morning Edition.*